The Social Brain

The Social Brain

Sociological Foundations

Sal Restivo

LEXINGTON BOOKS

Lanham • Boulder • New York • London

Rowman & Littlefield
Bloomsbury Publishing Inc, 1359 Broadway, New York, NY 10018, USA
Bloomsbury Publishing Plc, 50 Bedford Square, London, WC1B 3DP, UK
Bloomsbury Publishing Ireland, 29 Earlsfort Terrace, Dublin 2, D02 AY28, Ireland
www.bloomsbury.com

Published by Lexington Books
An imprint of The Rowman & Littlefield Publishing Group, Inc.
4501 Forbes Boulevard, Suite 200, Lanham, Maryland 20706
www.rowman.com

86-90 Paul Street, London EC2A 4NE

British Library Cataloguing in Publication Information available

Library of Congress Cataloging-in-Publication Data

ISBN 978-1-66692-705-4 (cloth ; alk. paper)
ISBN 978-1-66692-706-1 (electronic)

Dedicated to my wife Ya Wen

Contents

Acknowledgments

This book is for Jennifer, Wenda, Monica, and Lia, and for Leslie Brothers. Without Leslie this book would not have been possible. Leslie introduced the modern concept of the social brain into the neuroscience literature in 1990 and tutored me in all things brain and mind for several years in the 1990s in Santa Monica, California, and over email. Mario Incayawar, the first traditional Incan healer to earn a medical degree, has been a friend, colleague, collaborator, and teacher for many years since we first met as holders of endowed chairs at Harvey Mudd College in 2002. He; his wife, linguistic anthropologist Lisa Bouchard; and their daughter Sioui, a neuroscientist, have all contributed to my education as a student of mind and brain. Ellen Esrock and Linnda Caporaeal, friends and colleagues at Rensselaer Polytechnic Institute for many years, engaged my ideas on mind and brain with their own innovative insights and provocations. The late Mary Douglas was kind enough to entertain my early wanderings in the landscape of the brain and introduce me to Max Planck Institute neuroscientist Bob Turner, who encouraged my theoretical directions. Hélène Mialet was a late and critical addition to the list of my interlocutors on mind and brain. Special thanks to my next door neighbor and friend Katie, who allowed me to interview her four-year-old brain twenty-two years ago. And finally, Sabrina Weiss, friend, graduate student, and collaborator, wise in the ways of the life sciences and the life of the mind, helped me develop the first version of the social brain model, which I introduce in chapter 11.

Preface

Caveat Emptor

This book is about integrating the social self, the biological self, and the neuro-self. It is meant as a work of science and specifically as a contribution to sociological theory. Science in this context is understood in terms established by researchers in science and technology studies and the new sociology of science. These new fields emerged in the late 1960s and consolidated in the 1970s and 1980s. Their development challenged the classical view of science as pure, autonomous, self-correcting, and opening a window on unmediated objective reality. The naïve realist version of this perspective posited "the eye of the scientist," "things in the world," and "terms that refer." Scientifically prepared individuals looked into the world, saw things, and named them. That became the grounds for explaining them in causal terms and formulating equations and laws. The new history and sociology of science, more firmly grounded in empirical and ethnographic studies than previous research, demonstrated that science is socially constructed. It is the work of men and women working together in social, cultural, organizational, and ecological networks and contexts that unfold in history and across cultures. The individual "eye" of the naïve realist is a fabrication. There is no such eye, only culturally mediated perspectives.

The achievements of science are contingently objective. Thus, this book is not scientific by itself; I am not a scientist by myself. It is science and I am a scientist only in the context of its and my places in the unfolding of the linked generations of scientists collectively and intersubjectively testing ideas, theories, and experimental results. At the end of the day, I am an experiment, my book is an experiment, and my claims are an experiment. However certain I am of their truth, this is ultimately a collective decision of the evolving scientific community.

We can and do know things, but we do not know facts of the matter with absolute certainty. All facts of the matter escape their evidence and must be considered highly presumptive, corrigible, and fallible. We can and should be confident about what we know, but we should not allow what we know to be contaminated by absolute conviction. Science, like everything in the universe, including selves, bodies, and brains, is in flux, in becoming (*cf.* Bohm, 1957: 164; and Connolly, 2002: 15). Life, the universe, and everything are systems. Systems can be more or less open or closed. Open systems exchange information and resources across their boundaries; the boundaries of closed systems are impermeable. There are no perfectly closed systems. However, a system has to have a certain degree of closure if we are going to have reasonable expectations about revealing the causes and effects of actions in that system. We have to construct approximately closed systems in laboratories or identify approximately closed systems in the natural world to identify patterns and regularities that we might be able to formulate as "laws." The hypotheses and laws of the laboratory or the natural world must then be tested in the world of our experience itself. The complex open systems in nature yield to our inquiries only to the extent that they are closed. The solar system is such a system, complexly open but closed enough to allow us to figure out how to send humans and robots to the moon, Mars, and beyond.

Everyday life has levels of closure without which life would be impossible to navigate or to study scientifically. It would be impossible to do this if our lives were constantly uprooting our expectations. Imagine if the streets we cross randomly and often opened up sinkholes or were hit by earthquakes. These and other dangers are rare enough occurrences and so we can act and react predictably in and to life's circumstances and challenges. From a classical philosophical and some social theory perspectives, no definitive descriptions and prescriptions of reality are possible. We certainly don't have access to such descriptions and prescriptions in terms of "reality in itself," the *Ding an sich*. However, the levels of closure in our everyday realities mean that definitive descriptions and prescriptions-in-practice are possible.

This book is also a work in sociology. More specifically, it is a work in sociological theory and synthesis across the social, life, and neurosciences. I understand and practice sociology as a science. Many sociologists, other scientists, and journalists still question the scientific status of sociology. But it is recognized as a science by the US National Science Foundation and other private and public funding agencies around the world. Sociology is not easy to understand. It may seem to be a matter of common sense and introspective transparency, but that is a complex fallacy grounded in the folk sociology of everyday life. Social life requires a folk sociology that provides us with low-level theories about the hows, whys, whats, and wherefores of everyday life. This folk-level theory grounds our understanding of the symbolic, gestural, postural, cognitive, emotional, and behavioral repertoires that constitute our cultures. Folk sociology is not the same as professional sociology any more than the folk physics of alphabet blocks, Legos, and billiard ball collisions is anything like professional physics. It is therefore necessary for me to prime your sociological imagination as a foundation for understanding the sociology of the brain.

I have devoted my entire career to the sociology of the hard cases. The original hard case in the sociology of science was scientific knowledge itself. Classical sociologists of science and knowledge did not believe that scientific knowledge was rooted in social life. It existed outside of time, space, history, and culture. There could be no sociology of $2 + 2 = 4$. There were adumbrations of a sociology of scientific knowledge, mathematics, and logic in the classical period during which sociology crystallized into a distinctive discipline, a process that began in earnest during the 1840s. It was not until the emergence of science studies and the new sociology of science that those adumbrations could be forged into a sociological approach to scientific, mathematical, and logical knowledge (Bauchspies et al., 2006; Restivo, 2022; and see Collins, 1992, and Restivo, 2017). I've engaged all of these hard cases during my career and, beginning in the 1990s, I added the hard cases of the brain and God. In each case I am obliged to do two difficult things at the same time; explain sociology and show how it applies to the hard case. This is the rationale for devoting so much space to foundational chapters on the sociological perspective which constitute the scaffolding for the social brain model.

Introduction

The road to the social brain model will take us through the first ten chapters. These chapters are designed to construct the scaffolding on which it will be possible to construct a cohesive, comprehensible social brain model. Since that road will be long and winding and may challenge the tolerance of the reader who wants to get to the meat of the matter quickly and painlessly, I briefly sketch the rationale for the particular road I have chosen. But first some history and context.

This book appears in the wake of one of the major paradigm shifts in brain-theoretic science, the neuroscience turn of the late twentieth century (Littlefield and Johnson, 2012). Some earlier examples of paradigm shifts in brain-theoretic science include decoupling the brain from its connections to theological, scholastic, and mystical considerations in the sixteenth century (Bell, 2012); the new ways of thinking about the language of brain and self-hood in the United States in the 1840s (Morison, 2012); and a variety of brain paradigm shifts associated with twentieth-century poststructural philosophy and postmodernism (Gotman, 2012). In the latter context, neuroscience became a translational discipline. That is, it became a science that was translated for lay and science audiences, a translational process that stimulated efforts of the various audiences to speak to each other across disciplinary divides. This led to one of the many tensions my book is implicated in. That tension opposes neuro-reductionism to sociological reductionism. "Neuro" classically identified a hypothetical location—variously, the nervous system, the neuron, and the brain—that was the place to look for answers to humanity's deep questions about consciousness, the self, God, and the universe, locations that have turned out to be chimeras. On the sociological side, "the social" became a concept that seemed to reduce everything to a social construction. This side of the tension was based on a misunderstanding of social construction as mere representation and linguistics and implying relativism. "Neuro"-reductionism was for this reason a more serious concern, a reductionism that made all the other sciences uncritical consumers of neuroscience

(Littlefield and Johnson, 2012: 7). One of my objectives here is to untangle this tension and defend sociology as a non-reductionist discipline which can make important contributions to understanding brain, self, and consciousness on its own terms and in collaboration with the neuro- and other sciences.

Many, if not all, of the sociological assumptions I begin with about brains, minds, bodies, selves, and consciousness are already in the literature and have been for some time. One of the most recent contributions to this literature illustrates this history (Franks, 2019; and see Pickersgill and Van Keulen, 2012). The problematizing of the neurosciences and the cognitive sciences has also been in process while I have been working on the sociology of the brain. In science and technology studies, several books and articles have appeared since the early 2000s, which I cite at various places in this book (e.g., Beaulieu, 2000). The 2010 meeting of the European Association for the Study of Science and Technology included a track (#19) on "Approaches to Neuroscience Objects and Practices" (Bruder, 2010).

Another example of how the neuro-turn has forced sociologists to pay attention to cognition and the brain in new ways is the work of Stephen P. Turner (2002, 2018). Turner's exemplary scholarship addresses a variety of issues and problems that arise at the nexus of the cognitive sciences and sociology. He is a magician in the field of philosophical sociology who can make us wonder about the very ideas so many of us take for granted, including the very ideas of "the social" and "culture." I don't agree with his level of skepticism about the achievements of the science of sociology, but we would be foolish to ignore his skepticism and the new paths he suggests we try. Like much of the other literature I am drawing attention to here, Turner's work shows us there is an unexplored and challenging landscape before us. His perspective is not one that would lead to the path I have chosen. I do not claim to be exhaustive here; most of the related literature is referenced in the following text. What they all demonstrate collectively is that what is innovative about my contribution to the neuro-social nexus is the extent to which I have weaved the complex tensions, conflicts, and collaborations at that nexus into a synthetic model of the social brain. These references are the tip of an iceberg of issues, problems, and tensions at the neuro-social nexus that concretize what in an earlier period we would have called a Zeitgeist. We are awash in an atmosphere of research and theory on neurons and genes enhanced by enriched-environment studies, epigenetics, neuroplasticity, mirror neurons, and complexity and connectionism that demand our critical attention as sociologists and a new mobilization of sociological resources in the effort to understand brains and behavior.

Chapters 1, 2, and 3 introduce the sociological imagination. In order to understand the innovations I bring to the social brain model, we have to understand the very idea of "the social." This idea is in one sense part of our everyday, taken-for-granted world, our "common sense." This is the world of folk sociology. On the level of professional sociology, the idea of "the social" becomes non-obvious and counter-intuitive. This is not unusual when we move from the folk level to the professional level in science. The folk physics of lifting boxes, colliding billiard balls, and building things with everything from alphabet blocks to ice blocks is one thing. The professional physics of subatomic particles, gravity, and string theory is something that everyday common sense cannot grasp. These chapters provide most of the sociological scaffolding we need to understand the social brain model.

Chapter 4 demonstrates what happens when we raise the folk sociology of the self to the professional sociology of the individual in society. When we do this, we find a non-obvious, counter-intuitive reality that embraces the fallacy of introspective transparency, the "I" as a grammatical illusion, and the myth of individualism. This reinforces the scaffolding we constructed in chapters 1–3.

Chapter 5 takes the folk sociology of the body into the professional sociology of the body in society and politics. By the end of this chapter we will have raised the common sense notion of what a body is to the professional sociology of the body as a social network with a social history and a social context. There is no more "a body" than there is an "I." This further reinforces the scaffolding for my social brain model.

Chapters 6 and 7 raise the common sense notions of "genius" and "creativity" as matters of individual genes, neurons, and "ineffables" to the professional level of sociology. I show why it is more realistic sociologically to transform the classic metaphor of the genius standing on the shoulders of giants to a new metaphor of the genius standing on the shoulders of social networks. The non-obvious, counter-intuitive concept of creativity is that it is a social network phenomenon and not a matter of individuals or individual brains. This idea is developed in brief case studies of Albert Einstein, Stephen Hawking, and John Coltrane.

Chapter 8 reviews what happens when we are stuck in a world of mythical "individuals," "I's," "bodies," and "biomedical brains." In this context, philosophers are empowered to create fairy tales about brains in vats and simulations. If we are going to understand the social brain model, we will have to make sure we have extricated ourselves from the rationales for these fairy tales and the theologies they often hide, sometimes in plain sight.

Chapters 9 and 10 lay down the final planks in our scaffolding prior to constructing the social brain model. Chapter 9 considers the nature and limits of research and development in robots and artificial intelligence. This research has been driven by the mythologies I identify in the previous chapters. This chapter is in some ways an extension of chapter 6. We will not be able to build robots that are emotional and conscious in the way humans are on the basis of the myths of individualism, "I's," and isolated biomedical brains. There is no guarantee we will be able to achieve these goals with sociology's help (but see Collins, 1992: 155–84). We will have to consider the nature, differences, and potentials of social robots, sociable robots, robots 'r' us, and robots as robots. In chapter 10, I collect my various remarks on consciousness and draw on the sociology and anthropology of consciousness literature to demonstrate the rationale for my remarks. I weave all of this into a final consideration of sociology's solution of the "hard problem" of consciousness.

We have now completed the scaffolding for constructing the social brain model, and that is now our objective in chapter 11. Chapter 12 draws out some of the more important consequences of understanding that our brains are social brains for our individual and collective health and illness. Finally, in chapter 13 I consider the nature and limits of bringing sociology into brain studies.

Chapter 1

The Sociological Imagination

C. Wright Mills (1959: 3–4), in defining the sociological imagination, wrote: "men do not usually define the troubles they endure in terms of historical change and institutional contradiction." They don't connect their everyday lives to the dynamics of world history and society. They are blind to the ways in which humans and society, biography, history, self, and world interact. The structural transformations behind their personal troubles are invisible to them. The sociological imagination provides the map that has guided my journey to the social brain.

Most books about the brain that you can buy in your local bookstore or online are based on philosophical, biological, psychological, cognitive, or neuroscience maps. These maps are consistent with traditional atomistic views of the individual, the body, and the brain. Sociology is not widely understood and its core findings are non-obvious and counter-intuitive. But it can be approached with less anxiety and uncertainty if you realize that we humans are all sociologists. We have to be to negotiate our social world. We all, indeed, have theories that guide our knowledge of and understanding about social life. For example, you need to know who is in your dating pool, whom you can marry, and why. There are different cultural rules and expectations about communication, language, posture, and dress codes depending on whom you are interacting with: parents, children, teachers, shop clerks, and so on. Most Americans and Europeans take for granted that when someone greets you and extends his or her right hand, the expectation is "shaking hands"; that expectation is rooted in a social theory. Different cultures have different theories that support their behavioral expectations. In folk sociology there are no clear distinctions between theories and expectations. Shaking hands is not common in Japan except in international business settings. People greet each other by bowing. A bow can be casual and informal, no more than a small nod. Deeper and longer bows are more formal and used as signs of respect. If a greeting takes place on a tatami floor, a thick mat of woven straw, people get on their knees to bow. Bowing can convey thanks, an apology, a request, or asking for a favor. The custom of bowing with your palms together at chest level is common in Thailand but not in Japan. You have to have a theory about how time and space are organized in the everyday world so you'll know what time to wake up in order to get on the subway in time to get to your 9:00 a.m. class or job, or how, where, and when to apply for social security, unemployment insurance, or welfare benefits. We "present our selves" in different ways in different situations (Goffman, 1959), and we see our selves in part through the way others see us. Cooley (1909; and see Jacobs, 2006) describes this phenomenon as "the looking glass self."

The social theories that guide you through your everyday life are part of a folk sociology. You also carry with you a folk physics that guides you when you lift and carry things or build forts with alphabet blocks or Legos, ice blocks, or bricks and mortar; a folk chemistry guides your food preparation and eating habits; and a folk psychology guides your everyday engagements with emotions and thoughts. Each of these folk sciences can be upgraded by years of study into professional sciences such as physics, chemistry, biology, psychology, and sociology. Sociologists look more deeply and more analytically into social life than you have to in order to survive in your everyday world. By looking into social life scientifically sociologists are able to discover patterns of social interaction and the laws that govern the way groups of all kinds and sizes function. This leads to a fundamental understanding as well as the knowledge to guide public policy. Such research can overturn unexamined assumptions with important societal consequences. For example, the doctrine of separate but equal schools, a cultural norm in the United States for decades that was supported by Supreme Court decisions, was challenged in the famous case of *Brown v. Board of Education* (1954) and affirmed based in part on sociological studies. I discuss the details of this case below.

WE ARE ALL SOCIAL THEORISTS

Social theory is a basic survival skill. Experiences in organizations that have the same or similar structures and functions—private schools and public schools, for example—might lead to the observation that they have different rules of behavior. Going from classroom to lunch might involve an unruly group of boys and girls skipping, running, and walking in a carefree manner. The same activity in another school might find boys and girls lined up in separate lines and marching off in a teacher-imposed rule of silence. A child aware of these differences might wonder, "Why the difference?" The sociologist Charles Lemert's son, Noah, had an experience like this and eventually figured out that schools have "arbitrary" social rules like silence and segregated sexes because they are as much and maybe more concerned with civil discipline as with learning. Noah had developed a social theory within folk sociology. As we mature into young adulthood and come to know the world, we become increasingly able to state social theories about everyday social life in ordinary language (Lemert, 2021: 1–2). Ordinary social life is carried out by more and less socially skilled humans monitoring and trying to predict what the people around them are doing, intending, or expecting.

Understanding the facts of social stratification (that is, class differences, inequalities in access to the resources required for survival, and inequalities in power) leads to the conclusion that social institutions are designed to conceal the grounds of these differences and inequalities. Society is characterized by imposed illusions that mask the most powerful people consolidating, concentrating, increasing, and sustaining their power without being troubled by the complaints of their "subjects," from slaves and peasants to wage slaves.

The better we become as social theorists, the more power in knowledge and understanding we can achieve. We should pay attention to professional theorists because they spend more time studying society, are more focused and methodologically rigorous in doing this, and can generate more complex and sophisticated theories than folk sociologists. Some novelists and other intellectuals can do this, often with less theoretical sophistication than professional sociologists, by virtue of their training as more or less rigorous observers of social life. In some cases, their strong observational and communication skills can lead to significant insights, some the professionals might miss or not capture with as much depth and elegance. One thinks here of the skills of a Balzac or Dickens, a Virginia Woolf or Jane Austen.

As folk social theorists, we all consider ourselves experts on questions of everyday social life. But in reality, folk sociology is rarely able to overcome our lack of awareness about social structures and institutions. Collins and Makowsky (2010: 1) show why we must be skeptical and cautious about our folk sociologies. Our ability to negotiate everyday life requires a folk sociology, but these theories cannot penetrate the more fundamental mysteries of the social world. This is complicated by the Dunning-Kruger effect (Kruger and Dunning, 2000), a cognitive bias whereby people with limited knowledge or competence in a given domain greatly overestimate their own knowledge or competence in that domain relative to the known matters of fact or to the performance of their peers, people in general, and/or professionals. Some researchers also include in their definition the opposite effect for high performers, their tendency to underestimate their skills and knowledge.

All cultures have features their people take-for-granted, features that go unquestioned in everyday life. Sooner or later, all cultures produce thinkers who question and otherwise challenge those features, thinkers who become myth busters and debunkers of the illusions of everyday life. They do this by discovering and making us aware of ways of life in cultures from different places and times, ways of life that differ from our own. Lifestyles and life chances differ across social classes, age groups, sex and gender, and ethnicity. It takes serious research to uncover what goes on behind the closed doors where economic and political policies and deals are constructed. In this way sociologists reveal the invisible web of rules and institutions that influence (program) our behaviors, thoughts, and emotions more and less directly. Families, schools, and churches deliberately distract us from the realities of social power and forces. Sociology is one of the latest contributions to this discovery process. One of the best examples of the sociologist's ability to uncover the hidden realities of social stratification is John Porter's (2015) landmark study of social and ethnic inequality in Canada, a study originally published in 1965.

Things are not so simple. Intellectual life in all societies is primarily supported by the most powerful social classes and tends to support their interests. Sociologists are not immune to this principle. But the complexities and contradictions that characterize the societies which gave birth to sociology means that sociologies developed in conjunction with conservative, reformist, and revolutionary sectors of society. I come from the more radical streams of sociology that trace their origins to thinkers like Karl Marx and Peter Kropotkin. This is also the most realistic and objective tradition in the sense that to be radical means to get to the root of problems, pressing forward, ever forward, under the banner of the query "Why?" Radicalism defines the best form of science, an activity that does not find comfort in conclusions, views all answers as provisional, and is ever prepared to discard matters of fact in the face of new evidence (Hayden, 1967: 6). One of the areas of the social world that has been shrouded in mystery for millennia is religion, the realm of the gods, and God.

Understanding Religion Sociologically

This is not a random topic chosen to illustrate sociological thinking. Religious and theological issues permeate the history of the philosophy and science of mind, brain, self, and body. It is an issue in research and development in artificial intelligence, a factor in the history of the concept of genius, and shows up in the current obsession with simulations. I will draw your attention to this problem as those topics come into view.

Our fundamental understanding of religion began to shift as sociology crystallized in the nineteenth century. This was fueled in part by the emergence of biblical criticism in the late seventeenth-century German Enlightenment, the rationalism of the European Enlightenment associated with the work of John Locke, and the development of theology as a "science" in nineteenth-century German universities (Barr, 2000; Barton, 2010; Purvis, 2016). Theoretical studies of religion in this period are associated with the contributions of Robertson Smith (1846–1894), Ludwig Feuerbach (1804–1872), and most notably Emile Durkheim (1858–1917). Smith's work signaled a movement toward understanding religion as a social phenomenon, Feuerbach introduced the anthropology of Christianity, and Durkheim crystallized a fully sociological theory of religion.

Just before World War I broke out, one of the first credentialed sociologists, Emile Durkheim, published a book titled *The Elementary Forms of Religious Life* (1912, originally in French). Durkheim (1912/1995: 226–27) helped us explain why the faithful are not irrational and why atheists are mistaken on this score. The faithful are not irrational for believing in a higher moral power and believing that they are subject to it and owe their better selves to it. There *is* such a power: society. The act of worshipping strengthens the ties between the faithful and their god. But that god is not a type of being or entity; it is a symbolic representation of society. So going to church and worshipping together strengthens the ties between individuals and their society.

God is real, but not in the way people generally believe. God is real symbolically, not materially or in the form of any being or entity, material or immaterial. God symbolizes society. Durkheim discovered that when believers worship God they are worshipping their own society, their community. This is in one sense non-obvious because it is not apparent to inquiring minds or worshippers. Believing is not stupid, it is not irrational, and it is not a delusion. Atheist arguments would make more sense if they understood that believers are victims of a mistake in reference. And insofar as atheism organizes a moral order, formally or informally, it is itself a religion. All of this may become more obvious if you pay close attention to what actually goes on in churches when people are worshipping and attending religious services.

First of all, worshipping and religious observance can be carried out by individuals in private. If this is the only way they practice their religion, their religious experience will be more spiritual and self-enlightening than if they participate in collective observances. By isolating themselves, especially if they do so for long periods of time as wanderers or hermits, they will tend to have visions reflecting the objects of belief they learned before they wandered off. Hindu wanderers do not have visions of the virgin Mary; Catholic wanderers do not have visions of Vishnu. Such visions will reinforce their beliefs and they will become convinced that they have entered into a special relationship with the object of their belief.

On the other hand, those who worship collectively, if they pay close attention, will notice that there is something that happens when people gather to worship. They experience a oneness with those around them that is easily mistaken for a oneness with God. They experience what sociologists refer to as collective effervescence. This is a shared feeling across the group of thinking and feeling the same thoughts and emotions, a kind of excitement or emotional contagion that serves to unify the group. This is generated and enhanced by sharing the same object of focused attention—usually a religious icon, like the cross in Catholic churches. Pay attention to the ways in which you prepare to go to worship, how you dress, what you anticipate about the other people you will encounter, the positive feelings you have about joining them. All of this is reinforced by collective singing or even just hearing a choir sing or chant. If you pay attention to these sorts of details, you should see that worshipping is more clearly about your relationship to those around you than about your relationship to God. And sociologically this makes sense because worshipping God is really worshipping your community. The thoughts, actions, and emotions shared while worshipping are felt like a force on the individual and reveal the intervention of the community. This is possible because we are socialized to share a language and the concepts and emotions expressed in that language. This unfolds in society as collective representations and collective elaborations. For the wanderer or hermit, these same processes are experienced on an individual level. Long periods of isolation enhance the feeling of oneness with God. One comes to experience an individuated self-focused effervescence.

Durkheim (1912/1995: 440) expanded his theory of religion to encompass logic. The shape of logic and the level of its systematization and elaboration have varied across cultures but have never been missing. Logics, like morals, evolve in intimate conjunction with each other and the evolution of societies. In this way, by identifying religion and logic as collective representations and collective elaborations, Durkheim inaugurated the sociologically grounded rejection of transcendence. God, logic, time, space, cause, and personality are socially constructed; they are constructed from social elements. This does not strip them of objective content and value. Indeed, their very social origin is a sign that they are grounded in the nature of things (Durkheim, 1912/1995: 17–18).

Our beliefs, our abstractions (even mathematics and logic) are rooted in everyday social realities, not Platonic realms of forms or religious heavens and realms of an afterlife. Karl Marx (1818–1883), who was not fond of the sociology of his time, was nonetheless an innovative sociological thinker. In one of his earliest contributions (Marx, 1844/1956: 104–5), he argued that scientific activity, the material of that activity, and the language in which the scientist thinks are all social. They are social because the scientist is *"active as a man."* This means that Marx's and our own existence are *social* activities. The nature and shape of our consciousness represent the living shape of our community. Notice how this mirrors Durkheim's theory that God represents society. Marx goes on to note that the activity of consciousness is an expression of our existence as social beings. The individual is a social being, and while we can analytically distinguish thinking and being, they are a unity. This can be read as an adumbration of Gilbert Ryle's (1949) theory that the mind is just the body at work.

Durkheim and Marx represent two of the founding moments of the ideas we shall encounter in the following pages that (1) humans emerge on the evolutionary stage always, already, and everywhere social; (2) consciousness is an eminently social phenomenon; and (3) the mind is just the body at work. You can follow modern updates of the theories of religion, the gods, and God inaugurated in the works of Durkheim, Marx, and other classical theorists in Collins (1992), Maryanski (2018), Restivo (2021), and Warburg (1989).

Notice again that what has happened in the history of the gods, God, and religions is that humans made a mistake in reference. They did not have the correct knowledge based on sufficient experience to understand the social cause of God and projected their experience of collective effervescence outside of the group based on an elementary orientation to identifying causes for experiences. This gave rise to transcendental and supernatural explanations that were mistakes in reference. They referred their experience to a supernatural level because they did not have the cultural and intellectual resources to refer it to its natural origin. Furthermore, this means that religion is not originally and in principle about explaining the natural order, and God is not a god of the gaps, filling in beyond the limits of what science or reason can explain. Creation myths are about the creation of societies, of nations.

Failure to understand the sociology of religion, God, and the gods accounts for the mistakes of the "New Atheists" (notably, the "Four Horsemen": Hitchens, Dawkins, Harris, and Dennett) and their theist opponents (Restivo, 2023). Religion, the gods, and God are not delusions. People are not stupid for believing in God. They are responding to eminently social phenomena at the heart of what holds societies together. The point of the criticism of religion is not to eliminate it but to ground it in reality as what it is—the glue of society, a systematization of the moral order of a society. The reality of religion is nowhere better revealed than in the way it works to hold communities together when disasters like tornados and earthquakes occur. The most important clue to this mistake in reference is the comparative study of religion and culture and what it reveals about the variety of religions, their inevitable roots in social structures, and the way they systematically change as societies change. The account I've given of the origin of religion and the gods here took hundreds of thousands of years to unfold as societies and their rituals evolved.

Some of my students, friends, and even some of my colleagues in sociology have questioned my efforts to correct the mistakes in reference at work in our traditional views of religion, the gods, and God. A classic answer to these questioners was offered by sociologist Peter Berger (1963: 174). Berger was also a Protestant theologian. The debunking, disenchanting sociologist is peddling "dangerous intellectual merchandise," he wrote. What right does he or she have to challenge the taken-for-granted beliefs of others who are more or less at peace with their worldviews? Why bother those who are not inclined to probe for deeper understanding? Why not leave them alone? How should we think about this problem?

Our Responsibilities as Scientists

We might consider this first from the perspective of the responsibilities and skills of teachers with respect to their students, and of parents with respect to their children. We don't talk to freshmen the way we address participants in a graduate seminar. We don't talk to children the way we talk to adults. One of the most enlightening exercises I was asked to carry out in college was to choose a concept from my major and explain it to a six-year-old, a twelve-year-old, an eighteen-year-old, and a forty-year-old. My major was electrical engineering; I chose the vacuum tube (it was the 1960s!). The professor wanted us to understand explanation in relation to experience.

It is not so easy to break through the taken-for-granted features of everyday life. They tend to be solidly rooted and not easily shaken. So students will not throw their beliefs overboard upon hearing them critically undermined. The only chance that they will throw their beliefs overboard and embrace yours is if they continue to engage your ideas over and over and become increasingly immersed in your culture. Consider the classic sociological study of Bennington College students that began in 1935.

Social psychologist Theodore Newcomb and his colleagues carried out a classic study of Bennington College students, following them for years starting with their freshman year in 1935. The college in that era had a reputation for being a politically liberal campus. The college is expensive and attracts the children of wealthy conservative families. In the late 1930s, nearly 70 percent of these families were affiliated with the Republican party. As the 1935 class progressed through their education at Bennington, they became increasingly liberal. In the 1936 presidential race, almost 70 percent of parents favored the Republican Landon as opposed to the Democrat Roosevelt. A little more than 60 percent of the Bennington freshmen also favored Landon over Roosevelt. A little more than 40 percent of the sophomores favored Landon, and only 15 percent of the upper class favored the Republican candidate. Newcomb described this in terms of choices related to competing reference groups—conservative families and liberal students and faculty. The students' liberalism represented a pragmatic adjustment to their immediate social environment. Those students who remained liberal in their post-Bennington lives stayed connected with liberal reference groups—friends, husbands, and communities. By 1960, those Bennington graduates who had married conservative husbands and moved into conservative neighborhoods had shed their college liberalism for the values of their new conservative social environments. Newcomb noted that we tend to select reference groups compatible with our attitudes and values, but we can gravitate to reference groups that do not reflect our attitudes and values, and if we stick with them, they will redirect our attitudes and values (Newcomb, 1943; Newcomb et al., 1967).

Berger points out that students might avoid following through on the implications of their professors' claims and view them as an intellectual game. Play the game while in the course and then leave it behind as an interesting experience at best. This is a different way of thinking about reference group behavior. What justifies the liberal or radical (read: "scientific") agenda of sociology? Berger (1963: 175) maintains that liberal education is associated with intellectual liberation. This assumption does not apply to technically and professionally focused education (an assumption that we might consider challenging). Where it does hold, sociology (and science in general) is justified by the belief that consciousness is better than unconsciousness and that freedom depends on consciousness. I am at one with Berger in assuming that the "civilized mind" in our modern era requires contact with critical scientific disciplines, including sociology. Coming in touch with sociology in this context will make you a little less stolid in your prejudices, a little more careful in your commitments, and skeptical about the commitments of others.

In my own teaching at the college level, in order not to overwhelm the worldviews my students came into class with, I described my class in terms of opening a window that would allow them to look out on what sociologists were up to. We would observe them the way we would observe people in a new culture, one we wanted to learn about but not one we wanted to adopt as or incorporate into our own. Of course, it is inevitable that students will experience some degree of culture shock and come away from the experience, depending on what they brought to it based on prior experience, drawn to sociology or repelled by it—at least temporarily.

Sociology, Public Policy, and Social Activism

The doctrine "separate but equal" constitutionally sanctioned laws designed to achieve racial segregation by means of separate but equal public facilities for African Americans and whites. It was legally sanctioned by the Supreme Court's decision in *Plessy v. Ferguson* (1896). The Court ruled that the protections of the 14th Amendment applied to political and social rights (e.g., voting and jury duty) but not to social rights (e.g., sitting in the railroad car of your choice). The doctrine was first challenged in 1849 before the Supreme Court of Massachusetts. The U.S. Supreme Court subsequently affirmed the doctrine in 1908 (*Berea College v. Kentucky*) and again in 1927 (*Lum v. Rice*). In *Gaines v. Canada* (1938), *McLaurin v. Oklahoma State Regents* (1950), and *Sweatt v. Painter* (1950), cracks began to appear in the doctrine. The Court finally ended the doctrine of separate but equal in 1954 (*Brown v. Board of Education*). The Court's decision is notable for relying in part on the sociological research of Kenneth and Mamie Clark and other social scientists demonstrating that separate facilities were not in fact equal. The facilities, resources, and teachers for black students met lower standards than those for white students. Furthermore, segregation on the basis of race left African American students with enduring feelings of inferiority about their social status.

Another example of the practical application of sociological knowledge and understanding that is less impactful than *Brown v. Board of Education* but nonetheless of interest is the work of sport sociologist Harry Edwards (1942–) as a consultant to the San Francisco 49ers football team and the Golden State Warriors basketball team. Edwards designed the Olympic Project for Human Rights, which provoked the Black Power protest salute by African American Olympians Tommie Smith and John Carlos at the 1968 Summer Olympics in Mexico City.

One social science, economics, has dominated in the public policy arena in the United States and elsewhere. Sociologists are taken more seriously abroad, are active as public intellectuals, and regularly serve in public offices and even as presidents (e.g., F. H. Cardoso, president of Brazil, 1995–2003). Economists can tell us a lot about the statistics of wages and employment, but we have to turn to sociologists to understand how people experience the work world, whether employed or unemployed. Sociology's reputation suffers in America because the culture is dominated by the myth of individualism; a low level of compassion in the culture that is reflected among government officials who oppose safety nets such as Medicare, social security, and universal health care; and a history of anti-intellectualism.

CONCLUSION

Folk and Professional Sociologies in Conflict and Cooperation

The continuities between folk and professional sociologies can lubricate communication between professionals and the lay public. On the negative side, superficial examination of those continuities can lead to the idea that sociology is nothing more than common sense draped in fancy language that mimics science. But common sense is often contradictory; is it "birds of a feather flock together" or "opposites attract"? Common sense ideas about everything from "cheating" welfare mothers to the "free" market are contradicted by systematic sociological research. Some of the common sense notions that have been held over the centuries and that have been shown to be false by sociological research include that men are more intelligent than women, married people are happier than single people, people who commit suicide are mentally ill, and women have a maternal instinct to birth and rear children. My work as a sociologist will seem less alien to you if you appreciate the continuities linking folk and professional sociologies critically.

Coda: The Discovery of Society

Restivo (2018; and see Collins, 1992 on non-obvious sociology) is a biography of the concept of "society" sui generis. Society as a level of reality that could be studied scientifically crystallized in the middle of the nineteenth century in Europe in the work of Durkheim, Marx, Weber, and others. This book demonstrates the non-obvious explanatory power of sociology in chapters on the self, love, mathematics, religion, robots, the physics-mysticism nexus, the brain, the economy, and education. Collins and Makowsky (2010) explore the lives and ideas of the social thinkers who have shaped and continue to influence traditions in sociology. Focusing on the great names in the field, they weave biographical and conceptual details into a tapestry of the history of social thought in the nineteenth and twentieth centuries. And finally, Sydie (1987) examines the work of the classical social theorists (Durkheim, Weber, Marx, Engels and Freud) from a feminist perspective. Her focus is on the theoretical approach adopted by each theorist in his examination of the nature of human nature and, more specifically, the nature of sex relationships. In general, the dichotomized, hierarchical view of sex relationships common to each of the theorists forms the framework for her discussions and critiques.

Chapter 2

Sociology Comes into View

Sociology has been my tyrant. To paraphrase Freud (1895/1954: 119–120): A man like me cannot live without a hobby-horse, a consuming passion—in Schiller's words, a tyrant. I have found my tyrant, and in his service I know no limits. My tyrant is sociology; it has always been my distant, beckoning goal, and since I hit upon the hard cases of scientific knowledge, mathematics, logic, the brain, and god, it has come so much nearer. And with this came an understanding of the centrality of the myth of individualism in American culture (Barlow, 2013; Callero, 2013).

I was primed for the interdisciplinary and multidisciplinary waves that impacted the academic and professional disciplines during the latter half of the twentieth century. I was from the beginning an interdisciplinary sociologist and more European in my perspective than American. That means that I took Marx as a sociologist more seriously than did American sociologists in general, and that I was less contaminated by the psychological thinking rampant among American sociologists and a widespread prejudice among them favoring biological forces working in conjunction with or dominating sociological forces. European sociologists had a more robust sociological imagination relatively uncontaminated by psychology and the myths of individualism and free will by comparison with their American counterparts.

As a sociologist of science and mathematics I was never far from the frontiers of developments in the sciences. One of the key developments during the late twentieth century was the explosion of research and public interest in the neurosciences. My decades of work on the sociology of mathematics had persuaded me that mathematics did not come from individual mathematicians per se or from their brains. So why did they have brains, and what were those brains doing? When the neurosciences blossomed, I was ready. Even so, I wouldn't be surprised if you were skeptical and wondering what a sociologist is doing mucking about in the brain, and what could he possibly have to say about the brain? And more importantly, why would a sociologist's ideas about the brain be of importance to me? This book is an answer to that skepticism as well as to the curiosity that prompted you to pick up this book. Unlike most sociologists, I came to graduate school with a strong background in science. I had apprentice-level experience in engineering work from high school wood, metal, and electrical shops, and studied Maxwell's equations in one class and in the next class went to the working foundry that used to occupy one of the top floors of my school. After graduation, I worked briefly as a junior electrical engineer for the Seaberg Elevator Company in Brooklyn, New York. I spent four years as an electrical engineering major in college before switching to sociology, and I knew advanced mathematics, probability theory, and statistics. All of this reinforced my sense of myself as a scientist. My Marxist perspective inclined me to assume that sociology, the study of society and social relationships, was a science. Very few sociologists considered sociology a causal science, and this was even more the case for outside observers of sociology, especially physical and natural scientists and their philosophical allies and ideologues. This is still true to a large extent even though many decades of sociological research have helped to change some minds. This is not the case in other countries where sociologists play important roles in politics and policy.

In general, most critics of the scientific standing of sociology demonstrate little or no knowledge of the very best of advanced sociology. The National Science Foundation regularly funds fundamental research in sociology. In 2005, Dalton Conley became the first sociologist to win the foundation's Alan T. Waterman Award, awarded annually since 1975 to honor an outstanding young US scientist or engineer.

By the late 1960s, I was prepared biographically and professionally to contribute to the sociology of science but more importantly to the sociology of scientific knowledge. There are all sorts of issues that arise when science studies itself. These are beyond the scope of this chapter. What is important is that they are resolvable, and those of us who undertook this research task beginning in the late 1960s helped ground our understanding of scientific practice empirically for the first time.

My upbringing had sensitized me to the great differences between my life-styles and life chances and those of the wealthy. I think I became a candidate for Marxism when my dad took me to the shoe factory he worked in. I was ten years old. It was hard for me to get my head around the conditions under which he worked. The factory floor was dirty; the work space was dark, dusty, and had a strong chemical smell. I learned later that one of the sources of the smell was benzene, now a known carcinogen. I was especially struck by the pin-up calendars and nudie pictures pasted all over the walls.

The upshot of all this is that as a young adult I was already leaving behind traditional ideas about why we behave the way we do and why society is organized the way it is. It isn't on account of genes or neurons; biologists, physicists, and chemists couldn't offer satisfactory explanations (although they tried valiantly and arrogantly). It wasn't because of our individual characteristics; we weren't rich or poor because of certain personality traits. People didn't choose to be rich or poor. You weren't poor because you were lazy or unmotivated. And you weren't meant to play a certain role in society because you were a man or a woman, black or white, native American, Irish American, or an Italian immigrant. Social structures and culture mattered.

In the 1960s, the aerospace industry experienced a precipitous decline that left many highly educated, motivated engineers unemployed. The cultural climate of the time helped them to realize that you could be highly intelligent, college educated, and highly motivated and be unemployed. Class consciousness among these engineers led some of them to organize the Committee for Social Responsibility in Engineering and publish a magazine, *Spark*. Scientists and Engineers for Social and Political Action was organized during this period, and they published *Science for the People*. My own political awareness was awakened during my years at the City College of New York. Most of my professors in and out of engineering were left leaning politically. And the students collectively had a much more realistic understanding of society and social structures, race, class, and, to a lesser extent at that time, sex and gender as determining forces in our lives.

My humanistic concerns were constantly reinforced as my education unfolded. I became involved with Science for the People, the Dialectical Workshop, and the Radical Science Movement. In the end, I chose to work out my political agendas in the classroom and not on the streets.

I've often wondered why my radicalism was more voyeuristic, cerebral, and theoretical than expressed in activism on the streets. Perhaps it was because my mother kept me close to home, where I learned to entertain myself with whatever was at hand in our little land of love and poverty. While my dad was teaching me to box and defend myself, my mom was teaching me to be afraid of everything.

My parents were not political. My father had ideas about politics, but he didn't vote and he certainly didn't engage in public protests. He had some beef with FDR that I was too young to understand, and he was a constant critic of his union leaders. A colleague of mine told me that growing up on the Great Plains and riding on tractors all day across flat land that went on forever in all directions destined him for philosophy. Perhaps in a similar way, my home-bound upbringing destined me for theory work.

Sociology is a complex and diverse field, so when I say I am a sociologist I leave out important facts about what kind of a sociologist I am. I consider sociology a science, and a causal one. I leave no room for free will and precious little room for agency in human behavior. We are not automatons. We are open systems; our lives are not predetermined, but they are lawful. I doubt you'd have much trouble agreeing that as animal material organisms we "obey" the laws of physics, biology, and chemistry. To be clear, nature does not follow "laws" out of obedience. We and nature are subject to necessities by invariants, the "must-be-thus" (*so-sein-müssen*) of our universe. These invariants, universals, regularities, and patterns are imprinted with anthropomorphisms and moralities because of our human limitations, not because the universe is human, conscious, ruled by God, or moral. We are thermodynamic systems and reflect the laws (act in accordance with the "must-be-thus") of thermodynamics. As chemical systems we reflect the laws of chemistry. This should be obvious to many or all of you. But a majority of you I am sure would not be prepared to readily agree that we are also bound by the necessities, the "must-be-thus," of social systems. Don't worry, my sociology is not exaggerated science. I work within what is broadly understood to be "humanistic sociology," sociology with a human face, sociology concerned with issues of equity, compassion, and social justice. But I approach these issues as an advocate of a complex materialistic-critical realist worldview and a sociology that gives us laws of human and societal behavior. It's important to stress that we do not *obey* laws of physics, chemistry, biology, and sociology. We behave out of necessity.

Traditionally, when sociology has been grudgingly admitted to the sciences, it has been as a "soft science." It has often been devalued as "common sense" draped in sociological jargon. Sometimes it is conflated with or understood to be a form of social work, a helping profession. This is not the place for me to defend sociology as a science. I have done that in earlier writings that are listed in the bibliography. But everything I claim in this book is grounded in sociology understood as a causal science. Causality in complex systems is not the causality of billiard balls physics or balls rolling down inclined planes (*cf.* Bohm, 1957).

We are now ready to move forward and forge a path to a difficult goal for sociology: demonstrating how and to what extent society, social relationships, and social ties impact our brains. Don't be distracted by the fact that I've defined myself as a Marxist and an anarchist. Karl Marx was a brilliant philosopher and political economist but a sociologist in practice who understood that we are through and through social beings. Our selves are social; our minds and consciousness are social. His *Das Kapital* is not bogeyman literature. Marx offers detailed ethnographic studies documenting the everyday lives of working men and women along with profound theoretical considerations on the nature of capitalist society. Anarchism, as conceived by Peter Kropotkin (1842–1921), was a social science imbued with the evolutionary principles of cooperation and mutual aid (Kropotkin, 1908).

ENTERING THE LAND OF THE BRAIN
THROUGH THE GATES OF SOCIOLOGY

Beginning in the last decade of the twentieth century, the market place of ideas became flooded with books about the brain written by neuroscientists, biologists, philosophers, and science writers. Some were scholarly, some were popular introductions, and some were self-help books. What can a sociologist have to say about the brain that these authors haven't already said? To start with, sociology is not well understood by physical and natural scientists and philosophers, let alone public commentators and the general public. It is only in the last few decades that it has begun to gain some notice as a valid arena of research even among those who are not persuaded it is a science. Prominent conservatives like former Canadian prime minister Stephen Harper and political commentator George Will have urged, "Thou shalt not commit a sociology." Yet Will, who has a PhD in political science from Princeton, regularly seasons his witty and insightful commentaries with statistics that originate in the corridors traveled by sociological researchers. It is nonetheless true that sociologists are not commonly found in the United States among those writing about or being interviewed about the brain or other matters of public concern and interest. The British sociologist Hilary Rose has written quite a bit about the brain and neuroscience, usually in collaboration with her husband Steven Rose, a prominent neuroscientist. How do I come to write about the brain and with what standing?

It's important to keep in mind that beginning in about the middle of the last century the nature of disciplines began to change. Due in great part to the increasing complexity of the problems we were engaging at every level and in every corner of our existence as individuals and as a species, disciplines began to become more complicated. We started to talk about "multidisciplinary" approaches, "interdisciplinary" approaches, and even "transdisciplinary" approaches. By the end of the twentieth century, interdisciplinarity had embraced complexity and chaos theory, non-linearity, and fractal thinking. I came of professional age in formative years leading to that development. My intellectual biography prepared me more than most scholars to move into the flow of these movements.

Beginning in the late 1960s, a new interdisciplinary field began to crystallize: science and technology studies. This field was focused on the social origins and nature of science and technology. One of the most important things we did in the early years of science and technology studies was to study scientific practice up close. "Up close" meant going into laboratories and research organizations the way anthropologists go into the field and carry out detailed observations, distribute questionnaires, and do interviews. We invented the ethnography of science. Our reports about scientific practice in the physical and natural sciences, engineering, and mathematics revealed for the first time the actual practices of scientists at work. Up until this time, we relied on the recollections of senior scientists about their early work, scientific autobiographies which were idiosyncratic and psychological rather than socially and historically contextual, philosophers who wrote about what science should be, not what it was in practice, and journalists who followed the lead of philosophers and scientists as glorifiers of the work of science.

I emerged from this period with an interest in the sociology of mathematics. This was indeed a strange convergence. After I'd established a reputation in this field, a young Brazilian student was advised to come and study with me. When she went to apply for her visa, she was asked why she wanted to go the United States. "To study the sociology of mathematics," she said. The officer processing her documents spread his arms as far apart as he could and said: "Sociology? Mathematics? Impossible!" Her visa was denied. I had to write a letter to the Brazilian officials to inform them that there was indeed such a field of study even though it engaged only a handful of researchers. They gave her the visa.

A Feeling for the Social

Definitions of sociology are filled with words like "social institutions," which can make it sound like you're on your way to prison, and "social relationships," which may make you feel like you're tuning in to a dating site. To be good at something, to grasp it, you need to have a feeling for it. Evelyn Fox Keller (1983) titled her book about the Nobelist Barbara McClintock *A Feeling for the Organism*. This is something we find in great scientists. Einstein's most important attribute was not his rebellious anti-authoritarian attitude, a special genius for mathematics, or an encyclopedic knowledge of physics; it was his "feeling for the physical." He described it as akin to a religious experience or the experience of love. One has to develop a feeling of intimacy, of being "one with," the maize, in the case of McClintock; or the photon, in the case of Einstein; the rat facing a maze, in the case of psychologist Edward Tolman; the nature of the social, in Durkheim's case; and the concept of class for Marx. Definitions and books can't give you a feeling for sociology; that requires engaging and embracing it with all of your senses.

My goal in these early chapters is to help you develop a feeling for the social by taking you on my journey and allowing you to feel, touch, smell, hear, and see sociology along the way. McClintock could have handed you a cob of corn; Einstein would have invited you to ride a light beam in your mind. My way of introducing you to sociological thinking is more like Einstein's method than like McClintock's. Understanding what I mean by the social self and the social brain requires some understanding of the complexity of the sociological imagination. I have been slowly unveiling that complexity. As we continue, I will use words technical and commonplace designed to convey the colors and shapes, textures, and sounds of sociology. Given that this is coming to you through a text, how successful I can be will depend on a kind of osmosis, the process of gradual or unconscious assimilation of ideas, concepts, and knowledge. Let's take a wider look around against the background of what you've learned so far about sociology.

Think about moving through your days and nights. When you think about that, what do you see? Unless you are a recluse or in solitary confinement, you should notice that there are often other people (strangers as well as people you know) near you or around you. Think about whether those people are neutral parts of your landscape, like buildings and mailboxes, or they are impacting your behaviors, emotions, and thoughts in ways that are more or less invisible. I will bracket for the moment the possibility that buildings and mailboxes might be implicated in impacting who and what you are. Pay attention to the ways you react to the presence of others, especially to strangers you may bump into accidentally or ask for directions. Listen carefully to your conversations, which you will find often unfold in scripted, predictable ways. They involve taking turns, which requires that you recognize when someone is starting to come to the end of his or her remarks, at which point you can feel yourself getting ready to add your next remark. Watch the way you change your language, your posture, the way you dress when you are with your husband, wife, or lover; your dormitory roommates; the people at a party, a religious event, a wedding, a funeral.

Notice that when you are speaking to someone you are inclined to imitate their accent or speech pattern, even their posture. Think about how you feel standing in line waiting to get into a Beatles concert or a Mozart opera. Now think about how you feel inside the venue and why you feel one way and behave one way at the Beatles concert and feel and behave differently inside the Mozart venue. And notice that in both cases you feel differently than you felt waiting in line. Sociology at the end of the day is about elevating such everyday awareness (which you may have to be primed to pay active attention to) to a recognition that people play causal roles in constructing each other's behaviors, emotions, and thoughts. And as for buildings and mailboxes, consider that when you bump into a wall or drop a letter in a mailbox you get feedback that you are somebody, something, in the world. Even when you are alone, you will find yourself aware of others in your thoughts: memories of others, voices of parents admonishing or motivating you, rehearsals of forthcoming conversations, and so on.

On the assumption that all this sociology is common sense, consider the question of whether people who live together before marriage are less likely to divorce than people who do not live together. This question seems to have an obvious—common sense—answer. People who live together first will get to know each other better and have a better chance of making their marriage work. This is the common sense answer. Sociological research, however, shows that living together before marriage does not ensure that the couple will not divorce. Studying this problem in depth and over time brings out complexities that are not visible in the "obvious" answer. Eventually such studies clarified the contexts and circumstances under which relationships endure or end in divorce. The sheer number of people who cohabit before marriage means that people from different backgrounds and with different motives, values, and beliefs are involved. Think about these common sense proverbs: "birds of a feather flock together" suggests that the more alike people are the more likely they are to make a successful marriage, but "opposites attract" suggests the opposite.

The bottom line is that whether we are studying the behavior of heavier and lighter objects dropped from a tower or the cohabiting behavior of humans, we can't rely on common sense or the "obvious" for the correct answer. Let's be clear: common sense isn't what crazy people believe. It usually has some relationship to our everyday experience. So if *we* drop an iron ball and a feather from a tower, we can see that the iron ball reaches the ground first. But when we make this action a subject for research, we discover that they reach the ground at the same time in a vacuum. This leads to all kinds of interesting results about uniform acceleration, conservation of momentum, and so on that have implications for applied physics and engineering.

The same is true about sociological research, which often leads to counter-intuitive results in studies of human behavior that have implications for social policy. Our own personal experiences are a poor guide to the facts of the matter, as we will see in chapter 3 in the case of our relationship to our spinning Earth.

I grew up left out in the cold when it came to social relationships. I was obsessively drawn to social things but could not bridge the gaps. I once found myself in a small group of preteens playing spin the bottle. The "game" involves sitting in a small group, taking turns spinning a bottle, and kissing the person it points to when it stops spinning. I watched from a distance, rotating a small ball around a light bulb, pretending to think about planetary orbits but mystified about how to engage with the others. I remember riding a school bus and looking across the aisle where a middle school classmate had his arm around the girl he was sitting with and was squeezing her breast. They were both smiling at me. I had the desire to do that but no clue as to how to make it happen. It was that unbridgeable gap that disappeared virtually overnight once I had the basic tools of sociology at my disposal—social roles, social institutions, social change, social contexts, social networks, social,

social, social. And of course a little maturity and experience in the adult world helped me to develop in ways more sensitive to issues of race, class, sex, and gender. The fact is, however, that I never quite recovered from those early experiences which left me feeling marginalized throughout my life but with a greater sense of control than I'd had in my youth. I found value in being marginal and cultivated it.

Sociology pulled me in as deeply as it did because I had been left out of the game of society for so long and had become obsessively curious about people and relationships. Initially, it gave me a grip on things from a rational, logical, scientific distance. It took a long time, many years of schooling, and a broadening of my experiences in the world to make me a human being, a social being, with a sociological imagination.

The Social Brain Comes into View

The idea that your brain is and is part of a social network crystallized in the early 1990s (Brothers, 1990, 1997). But it did not overtake classical concepts of the brain as an independent, biomedical organ that was the font of all of our behaviors, emotions, and thoughts. A neuroscientific turn made the brain a center of interest in science, in the media, and in the public square. Countries around the world, including the United States, began implementing policy initiatives to stimulate research on the brain. In the United States, the first of these initiatives was President Bush's 1990 Decade of the Brain proclamation. In 2013, President Obama proclaimed the BRAIN initiative. Between 1990 and the first decades of the twenty-first century, other nations, from Saudi Arabia and China to Great Britain and the European Union, poured millions of dollars into brain research. All these initiatives were based on the idea that the brain was the causal source of all of our behaviors, emotions, and thoughts. This was the brain viewed through the lenses of biology, medicine, and the myth of individualism. The overwhelming bulk of these monies went to the neurosciences. There were some inter- and multidisciplinary perspectives that got some attention, such as the Brains in Dialogue workshops I participated in that were held in various venues between 2009 and 2011. These workshops even included sociologists and neurological patients. The funding for these efforts was dwarfed by the funding for research on the biological medical brain. At the same time that these programs were being put in place, a new way of thinking about the brain was developing. This new way of thinking about the brain was based on ideas about networks, connections, and interdependencies. This book is an introduction to that social brain concept and why it should matter to you and your health care professionals.

The road to the social brain paradigm has been laid down by social scientists working independently and in collaboration with life and neuroscientists (i.e., neurosociology) and by neuroscientists open to sociological consider-ations (i.e., social neuroscience). My work in this field has been guided by the sociological imagination. My approach deviates in important ways from early collaborations and cross-overs between the neuro- and social sciences. These collaborations and cross-overs have informed my work in important ways, but they tend to (1) be supported by a scaffolding that contains more and stronger biological and medical planks than sociological planks, and/or (2) fall short of the strong social constructionist perspective I advocate (e.g., Franks, 2019; Pickersgill, 2013; Pickersgill and Van Keulen, 2012; TenHouten, 1997).

I taught sociology to undergraduates and graduate students for about fifty years, and that experience taught me that it is extraordinarily difficult to plunge people into sociology and have them grasp what it's all about. The resistance I experienced made me realize that my views violated fundamental assumptions my students were bringing into my classes. My sociological per-spective was bumping up against core assumptions in American culture about what it means to be an individual. I encountered these assumptions all over the world in my teaching and lecturing travels, but they were more strongly embedded in American culture than elsewhere in the world.

One of my goals in this book is to illustrate the ways in which the new social brain concept should matter to you. It changes the basic ways in which we think about and approach the brain in health and illness. It contributes to solving what is known in some circles as the "hard problem" of conscious-ness. In order to achieve that goal I need to help you think sociologically. That is why my initial goal has been to travel sociological roads to get to the social brain highway.

Why not skip all of this preliminary material on the sociological imagina-tion and begin directly with the social brain paradigm or at least the "hard problem" of consciousness? One reason is that the audiences for this book, lay and professional, American and European, Western and non-Western, have been to varying degrees under the influence of the myths of individu-alism, free will, and brain- and gene-centric thinking. Another is that I've observed sociology starting to seep into the public arena through major media, including *New York Times* bestsellers, and failing to reach its mark. From *New York Times* writers David Brooks (2011) and Nicholas Wade (2009) to Pulitzer Prize–winning biologist E. O. Wilson (2012), sociological perspectives are beginning to reach a wider and wider audience. But these efforts fail to scale the wall of assumptions about the individual biological self. The result is that these authors and others like them bring a half-filled tool chest and reach incorrect or limited conclusions. We're getting close though and I want to use this opportunity to help push us over that wall and reach more robustly sociological conclusions. I can only achieve this in a concise elementary way at this point, but what I can convey of the sociological imagination will be enough to underwrite my perspective on the social brain. This is more important than ever now that we are in the landscape of mind, brain, and consciousness. As I alluded to in my introduction, the very idea of a social brain rests on the very ideas of a social self and a social body. These are neither transparent nor readily accessible to common sense. And indeed the myth of individualism is a serious obstacle we must overcome to communicate that we have social selves and social bodies, a prelude to understanding that we have social brains.

The Vulnerability of Free Will

Once upon a time in John Wayne's America I met a man about my age at a party. Let's call him Bill. Our lives had unfolded in much the same ways. Bill's story was the standard American self-made-man story. Poor childhood, uneducated parents, school and home environments poor in the resources for enriching young minds. And yet here he was a successful professional. He attributed this to his individual spirit, his will to overcome, his freedom to choose. His story was overrun with "I's": I did this, I achieved that, I chose, I was chosen, I was elected, and so on. And that's how I would have told my story had I not come to understand social construction, social contexts, social structures, and social networks. On the surface, it appeared that I had chosen to go into engineering freely. But "I" made this choice in the middle of a technological revolution driven by lofty visions of space travel. These visions, linked to the space race, the arms race, and the Cold War, were already beginning to spur my teachers and counselors to guide students good in math and science into applied science and engineering when *Sputnik 1*, the first artificial Earth satellite, was launched into an elliptical low Earth orbit by the Soviet Union on October 4, 1957. Five years later, on September 12, 1962, John F. Kennedy told an audience at Rice Stadium in Houston, Texas: "We choose to go to the Moon."

It was no accident that already in the mid-1950s my interests were evolving from dinosaurs and stamp collecting to engineering, rockets, and space travel. The government was pouring more and more funding into science and engineering education. Pamphlets and films were produced and made available to school guidance counselors that encouraged students to go into science, math, and engineering. Contemporary STEM (science, technology, engineering, and math) programs are an echo of those programs and follow the same principle of the "technological fix." "Technological fix" was coined in 1965 by Alvin Weinberg, one-time director of the Oak Ridge National Laboratory. Weinberg advocated for engineering innovation as a generic tool for solving technological problems but also problems commonly conceived as social, political, or cultural. As we will see in later chapters, we are now living in the age of the "neuroscience fix." Private industry got into the technology-fix act too. General Electric produced a series of comic books that featured scientists and engineers as heroes. These heroes didn't leap over tall buildings in a single bound or save damsels in distress from falling off sky scrapers. They invented things and solved problems in physics and math. One of these General Electric comics featured the electrical engineer Charles Steinmetz (1865–1923), "the wizard of Schenectady," home of General Electric.

Statistics show extraordinary growth in a variety of science indicators, such as the number of science articles, conferences, and degrees granted around the *Sputnik* event. The growth curves show a *Sputnik* "bump," a jump in many science indicators. All of this made it possible for me to go to graduate school on stipends, fellowships, and tuition free City College. On September 2, 1958, just as I was entering tuition free the City College of New York, President Eisenhower authorized the National Defense Education Act (NDEA). *Sputnik* spurred this act along with other science initiatives, including DARPA (Defense Advanced Research Projects Agency) and NASA (National Aeronautics and Space Administration). Even the social sciences benefited from these developments. My acceptance into graduate school came with a three-year NDEA fellowship in comparative social structures.

This wasn't simply a question of the government wanting to fund social science per se. As the Cold War heated up, the study of non-US and non-Western cultures became an issue of national defense and national security. The fellowship was designed to train social scientists to assist the government in their regime change and counter-revolutionary actions in the "Third World." When my NDEA funds were used up, the National Science Foundation (founded in 1950) chipped in to help me complete my PhD, again tuition free. And of course I was shoveled out of the regular public school system earlier and into the elite public school system focused on science, engineering, and mathematics.

It is fair to ask: Didn't an "I" have to play a role in taking advantage of the resources available in the various contexts I've described? Didn't "I" have to work hard in order to deserve the NDEA fellowship? This is a fair question and one I will have to let the rest of the book answer. It won't answer the specifics of my life story, but it will offer a general answer. It will come down to the counter-intuitive idea that the "I" is a grammatical illusion. We are all social in a radical sense, as opposed to being individuals in a radical sense. From birth to the present, contexts, structures, and networks have been shaping my thinking and my "choices," and yours too. This has implications for our age of identity politics, which I consider in chapter 13.

Whatever earlier social forces in my life had made me imagine myself as an astronomer on Mt. Palomar, as I progressed through grades 5–7 guidance counselors and science teachers funneled my interests into engineering. And their advice was being shaped by forces at work in the larger society. My friend Bill, without the benefit of a sociological imagination, was at the mercy of our culture's myths of individualism, individual initiative, and self-interest. His story was all about "I's"; my story was all about contexts, structures, and networks. His story was a small tale within the larger narrative of the Great Man theory of history. That theory claims that history is the result of the actions of Great Men, good and bad: President Lincoln freed the slaves, Gabrilo Prinzip started World War I by assassinating Archduke Ferdinand, Hitler caused the Holocaust.

The great Russian writer Lev (Leo) Tolstoy (1828–1910) proposed an alternative to the Great Man theory in his novel *War and Peace* (1869/1996). The closing pages are a treatise in the philosophy of knowledge, the nature of causality, and the illusion of free will. The Great Man Napoleon is portrayed as a baby in a carriage, holding a couple of strings and imagining he is driving the carriage. What actually propels the carriage are social, cultural, and historical forces. This will sound more reasonable and become more transparent as my narrative unfolds.

CONCLUSION

Remember *Ragged Dick* (Alger Jr.,1868/2017)? Unless you grew up in America and are around my age, the name may not resonate. You might be more familiar with his creator, Horatio Alger Jr. Ragged Dick, Richard Hunter, is Alger's "rags-to-riches" literary invention. It has become absorbed into the American mythos of the "self-made man." The curious thing about Alger's rags-to-riches boys is that their success depends in the end on the luck of finding wealthy businessmen mentors and patrons. Alger himself sponsored philanthropic efforts to help the Richard Hunters of the world. There were two female protagonists in Alger's writings, Helen Ford and Tattered Tom. Tattered Tom dressed and lived like a boy, and like many Alger heroes, she was a news boy. Girls are not prominent in Alger's writings because the possibility of finding a mentor or patron in the business world was not open to them.

The Horatio Alger myth of individual success through will and initiative is not just a myth about America, it is a myth about the Alger stories themselves. If you read my biography psychologically—or what is basically the same thing, from the perspective of the American mythos—it looks like the story of a strong-willed boy taking initiative and pulling himself up by his own bootstraps. To tell the story this way requires being blind to social forces. Go back and read the Mills introduction that opens chapter 1. This inability to see the social is a trained incapacity in the families, churches, and schools that "educate" us to think in terms of individuals, individual self-interest, and the rags-to-riches myth. This all unfolds in the context of the economic ideology of capitalism. Remember what you learned about opportunity and social mobility as part of the story of American exceptionalism? Social mobility rates are not substantially different in America than they are in any modern industrial nation-state. And they depend in any given era on political and economic structural factors that can raise or lower rates of social mobility. Incidentally, the phrase "pulling yourself up by the bootstraps" comes from an eighteenth-century fairy tale and was a metaphor for an impossible feat of strength. The American mythos transformed the phrase into a slogan of individual initiative and the ability of "any American" to become president of the United States.

The early phases of my story superficially support the Horatio Alger myth. The later phases show how a folk sociology that was visible to my peers finally started to come into view for me. I was then able to build on this as I went on to a professional transformation that opened up new vistas of understanding and explanation. Not all sociologists go as far as I did. But everything before graduate school primed me for taking the concept of social structure and running with it. Let the games begin.

Chapter 3

Evolution Invents the Social

WHO AND WHAT ARE WE?

As soon as we humans awakened in our African homelands (and perhaps elsewhere) we found ourselves haunted by three questions. At some point, before we developed languages, these questions must have sat in our awareness like a small, dense, black orb, troubling, mysterious, and out of reach. This image comes from a recurring experience I remember from infancy. The black, dense orb sat uneasily somewhere in the middle of my head. It seemed to want to tell me something. It made me feel uneasy, not anxious, not frightened. Eventually, we were able to articulate those questions: Where did we come from, who are we, and where are we going? Sometimes these questions blended into a plaintive "Why are we here?" And finally, "Why is there anything at all?"

History is awash with efforts to answer these questions, which early on came under the jurisdiction of philosophers and theologians. As the sciences evolved they haltingly added substance to the misty, mystery-laden, metaphysical, transcendental, and supernatural ideas of the philosophers and theologians. By the time Charles Darwin arrived on the scene, we were prepared to construct biologically grounded answers to these questions. Between Darwin and late twentieth-century neurosciences, these questions began to absorb social and behavioral scientists alongside the still strong voices of the philosophers, theologians, and physical and natural scientists. Already in the early years of the Age of the Social (1840–1930), the leaders of the embryonic social sciences understood our radically social nature. In the last thirty years or so that understanding has finally begun to make an impression across the sciences and has been slowly seeping into the public imagination. Given our cultural mythologies and predispositions it is not surprising that we are being exposed to the nature and significance of the social not by sociologists but by biologists, neuroscientists, and philosophers. The idea that we are social, and even that we are radically social, is not new. What is new is the stronger claim I make that we humans appear on the evolutionary stage already, always, and everywhere social. We do not arrive as individuals but as social animals. Social and cultural processes make us into individuals without ever overriding our essential social nature.

If you grew up in America and were educated in our public schools, you were, like me, overtly and covertly exposed to America's guiding myth of individualism. We were introduced to the exploits of heroic, iconic individuals who made history: George Washington, Abraham Lincoln, Teddy Roosevelt, FDR and Eleanor Roosevelt, Rosa Parks, Martin Luther King Jr. We were given mythical folk heroes to admire, like the superhuman lumberjack Paul Bunyan. The movies reinforced this myth, and some of us can at this moment conjure the image of John Wayne. Individualism also had its anti-heroes: Americans like Benedict Arnold, world figures like Genghis Khan, Napoleon, and Hitler. All of this expressed what was known to historians as the "Great Man" theory of history; that is, history can be largely explained by the exploits of "men" of extraordinary ability, intellect, and courage, and often with excessive capacities for violence. It was easy for me, as for others, to accept the "common sense" rationale for this idea because we experienced ourselves as free-willing individuals. We might not be capable of heroic acts or genocidal violence, but we could feel ourselves willing our way through the behaviors needed for basic everyday survival. Even in my first years as a college student, I extolled the virtues of what I saw as Great Men.

For reasons I don't remember clearly, Anthony Eden was one of the men I wrote favorably about in my journals. I was seventeen when ill health forced Eden to resign as the British prime minister. I was concerned at the time about what I saw as a decline of quality in leadership at all levels of society. I read Eden's resignation as the loss of a paragon of the great leader. It is clearer to me today why I wrote (somewhat naïvely) with awe about the heroic leadership of Churchill in war, politics, and letters. As my education proceeded and the scope and scale of my experience expanded—through travel and virtually by way of books and various media—my belief in myself as a free-willing individual began to wane. And then I read Tolstoy's (1869/1996) *War and Peace*. Tolstoy's *War and Peace* may be the most important epistemologically informed novel ever written. Tolstoy writes with great insight about what I later came to call the fallacy of introspective transparency. That is, everything about our own awareness, our consciousness, our mental acts seems to be absolutely clear and a reflection of our individual free will and agency. And then I read Tolstoy's description of Napoleon—a child holding a couple of strings inside a baby carriage and imagining that he is driving it, and moreover convincing others that he is driving the carriage. Now I began to think about the limits of experience.

The Fallacy of Introspective Transparency: Why We Can't Trust Our Experience

Consider that we experience the Earth as stationary. And yet we know it moves. It wobbles in precession on its axis, is rotating at any point on the equator at 1,000 miles an hour, travels around the sun at 66,000 miles an hour, and is part of a solar system orbiting about the center of the Milky Way at 140 miles per second. The Milky Way itself is part of a cluster of galaxies (the Local Group) traveling toward the center of the cluster at 25 miles per second. And the Local Group itself is speeding through space at 370 miles per second. We feel *none* of this complex system of motions. So if our experience deceives us, how do we know about all of these motions? We know about them because of the collective intersubjectively tested experiences of scientists working across many linked generations. If we are deceived by our experience in the case of the motions of the Earth, could we be deceived by our experience of our free will and agency? This is exactly what I claim: our individual experience fails us even in our most intimate, immediate, transparent sense of who and what we are.

Tinkering Our Way through Evolution

We are evolution's most radical experiment in social life and survival. Evolution is an extremely complicated multilevel, multidimensional process that operates on many different time scales. But it is driven by an overall paradigm. If we personify evolution as a certain type of scientist-engineer (let's call it E), we see E acting like a tinkerer. To tinker is to *attempt to repair or improve something in a casual or unfocused way.* The tinkerer experiments and embraces failures in trial-and-error operations. The tinkerer's goal is simply to succeed, to make something that works without thinking about immediate functions or long-term objectives. E thus works without a specific goal in mind, takes advantage of whatever materials are at hand, and tinkers them into something that works. We can characterize the main feature of E's work as marked by contingency. What resources are available in E's local environment that it can play with? And this indeed is the way ethnographers of scientific practice have characterized the day-to-day work of scientists (e.g., Knorr-Cetina, 1979). The idea of evolution as a tinkering process is associated with the work of François Jacob (1977).

Different tinkerers and the same tinkerer at different times will produce different solutions to the same problems. To give a specific example, consider that all living things share the same organic molecules and metabolic pathways. If E is a tinkerer, then we can assume that new functional proteins do not appear anew but arise from rearranging genetic elements. We see this reflected in the similar DNA sequences of fruit flies and pigs that cause wings to appear in one case and legs in another. E can be expected to work under the same natural constraints as humans and especially the law of limited possibilities. The law of limited possibilities is illustrated by the invention of the oar. Keep in mind that in this case the tinkerer is human and does indeed have an objective. Many different kinds of oars can be tinkered into shape. But they all must meet certain requirements, natural constraints, if they are going to power a boat. Oars can come in a variety of shapes, but they can't be constructed in any shape whatsoever. This principle operates in technology but also in culture more generally, and we can assume it applies in E's case too. Objects rationally designed by humans might in some cases be impossible to distinguish from the random exploration of a solution space (de Lorenzo, 2018). This shouldn't be strange since human rationality is the result of evolutionary processes. The processes of invention and discovery whether driven by E's tinkering or rational human intelligence must necessarily undergo multi-objective optimizations. We should expect to find similar relational logics guiding biological evolution and human design. And both processes will necessarily exhibit imperfections and less-than-optimal solutions. The results of "blind" tinkering E, amateur bricolage, or reasoned design may be indistinguishable. They all will follow different itineraries that lead to the same optimal attractors in a solution space.

What we find when we study science in practice is a collective generational process. Science *in practice* is contingent and opportunistic. Scientific practice involves using the results of earlier efforts to generate new results—everything from measuring devices and chemical reagents to test animals and mathematical equations. In a sense scientists make their own reality and test it progressively against the impositions and constraints of the world outside artificial and natural laboratories. This applies to theorists, too, whose theories are in fact experiments in logic, reason, and mathematics based on experimental evidence produced by research scientists. Theories are not idle speculations or wild, ungrounded imaginings. Scientists are not searching for "truth" in some abstract sense but for something that works. Their goal is success, not "truth" per se. This practice nonetheless leads to corrigible, tentative, fragile, and dynamic facts of the matter.

Evolution Invents the Social

E's tinkering leads to the discovery that cell proximity in primitive organisms is a survival mechanism. Keep in mind that E's tinkering results are produced in an arena ruled by the principle of natural selection: blind variation and selective retention (Campbell, 1960). More complex forms of "colonial cooperation" followed and led to the emergence of multicellular animals and internal fertilization among amphibia and reptiles. More advanced cooperation made its appearance among the mammals. The placenta, mammary glands, and long gestation and dependency periods added a strongly social dimension to the adaptation process. Increasingly among the primates and then humans the survival of the young became dependent on extended caring behavior by two, three, or more adults in a supportive community. Humans emerged as one of the eusocial species, building up dense complex social networks around the campsite. The campsite is the human equivalent of the nest in other species. In fact, cooperation operates on all scales of life, from genes and cells to societies (Gorney,1972: x, 46ff, 96ff; Wilson, 2012: 140ff). I discuss this further in chapter 11.

In summary, E's tinkering led to cellular collaboration, which eventually led to grouping behavior and sociation. The importance of grouping behavior is illustrated by the fact that a single prey is more likely to survive a predator's attack in a group. Sociation refers to the stable and patterned micro-level forms of more or less intense face-to-face interactions. Primary groups are small-scale, close-knit, face-to-face, long-lasting, intimate relationships. The nuclear family, close friendships, and short- and long-term relationships are examples of primary groups. Secondary groups can vary in size, last for various periods of time, and are characteristically impersonal. They tend to be task oriented rather than relationship oriented. The committee at your work place tasked with organizing a party is an example of a secondary group. A school committee organizing a bake sale is another example of a secondary group. Secondary groups can of course incorporate primary groups. Your entire family may get involved in planning the school's bake sale.

If we view life from an evolutionary perspective we find that most humans have lived in primary groups. Secondary groups proliferated as the industrial age unfolded. This process gave rise to classical primary-secondary dichotomies such as rural-urban, country-city, and the one best known to social scientists, Gemeinschaft-Gesselschaft (communal society-associational society; Aldous, 1972). Communal societies, typified by rural, peasant societies, are characterized by face-to-face relationships that are defined and regulated by traditional norms, values, and beliefs. These traditional regulatory "laws" of family, kinship, and religion are weakened in the associational society by the ideals and goals of self-interested rationality. There is a shift from personal, direct, face-to-face interactions and a sense of universal solidarity to impersonal and indirect, primarily economically and politically oriented interactions.

These interactions are embedded in processes of rationalization, bureaucratization, professionalization, specialization, mechanization, and commodification. These transformations generate feelings of alienation (Jaeggi, 2014; Neuhouser and Smith, 2018). The feeling of alienation is brought about by the loosening or destruction of primary ties. In the twentieth century, technological progress led to the development of technologically mediated relationships. The classical telephone conversation is a prime example of such a relationship. The digital revolution gave rise to more complex mediations.

Face-to-computer interactions are a key mediation in the digital technological revolution. This transition from primary and secondary relationships to complex technologically mediated relationships has profound implications for the human condition. Face-to-face relationships are a crucial feature of human evolution. They are the basic means for communication and the emergence of consciousness, mind, and emotions. We can view mediated relationships as a danger to this evolutionary construction or as a new stage in the evolution of relationships, communications, and emotions. Are we witnessing the emergence of new human-machine species—cyborgs or machine species that will compete with fleshy humans for an ecological niche? The digital revolution can be viewed as an existential threat to the human species or a "natural" evolutionary development, another tinkering context for E. Perhaps we are on the verge of a new "Great Leap Forward," such as the one that characterized the Upper Paleolithic Age forty thousand years ago. We are faced with many unknowns as we move through the digital age at the same time that humans and other species, along with the planetary ecology itself, face doomsday possibilities. Whatever our future holds in store for us and our planet, it should be clear that messing with face-to-face relationships portends radical changes in our communicative, mental, and emotional lives (Dunn, 2021; Restivo, 2022: 301–24; Sykes, 2020).

Humans have always had access to mediated communication (from drumbeats to smoke signals). But the key moments in the evolution of mediated communication are associated with the emergence of literacy. One of the key moments in premodern times was the invention of the printing press by Johannes Gutenberg around 1440. Woodblock printing was available in China at least as early as the Han dynasty (206 BCE–220 CE). The Chinese also invented movable type around 1040 CE (attributed to Bi Sheng).

In our global village, people often find themselves or their organizations engaged in cross-cultural settings. These settings are replete with potential ambiguities due to variations in gestural, linguistic, emotional, and postural standards. Face-to-face relationships are much more reliable in such ambiguous communication settings which involve cooperation, conflict, and negotiations. There are professionalized international networks in which a great deal can be accomplished through virtual modes of communication aided by high levels of standardized technologies and symbols. This is true for example in the airline industry. But to return to the other horn of the dilemma, we know that face-to-face interactions and grooming behaviors are important aspects of non-human primate behavior. Among infant macaque monkeys, for example, the more face-to-face interactions they have with their "mothers" the more sociable they are in later life. The relevance of these studies which show long-term sociability effects of face-to-face interactions is that humans and macaques, for example, exhibit similar child-rearing behaviors and developmental trajectories.

Self, Society, and the Digital Dilemma

We are facing a digital dilemma. The development of multilevel, mediated relationships and communication platforms has produced increasingly prominent and pervasive alternatives to face-to-face relationships and communicative modes of interaction. The dilemma is this: on the one hand, what we might call "tertiary" modes break down geographical and temporal barriers to face-to-face interaction. It is now possible to put yourself instantly and efficiently in contact with anyone anywhere in the world with an internet connection. On the other hand, tertiary modes, at least two steps removed from primary relationships, cannot reproduce the ways in which face-to-face relationships support gestural, voice modulation, postural, and emotional options. These are not just basic ingredients of communication. Face-to-face interactions engage more of the senses than tertiary interactions. They are the primitive origins of and sustaining factors for consciousness and emotions. To put it differently, primary, secondary, and tertiary modes are associated with different types and states of consciousness and emotions.

Consciousness and emotions are relational; they are in-between phenomena and not phenomena that are generated and sustained within the individual. So the digital revolution is leading to new forms of consciousness and emotions—not face to face but face to interface. We can misinterpret meaning and intent in face-to-face interactions, but digital forms of communication tend to reduce the number of factors available for interpretation and so the possibilities for miscommunication are greater. This is not simply a matter of managing interpersonal and organizational communication; it comes down to a process that arose in the evolution of animal life and that is implicated in the biology and sociology of survival.

Looked at from the vantage point of the evolutionary stage, what we have are variously mediated forms of relationships and communication competing for ecological niches and for survival. Evolution, we've seen, unfolds on multiple levels, in multiple dimensions, and on multiple time scales. One can imagine that a species heavily based on mediating technologies (robots, for example) might have better long-term survival potential than humans. These are the considerations being discussed and debated around ideas such as "the singularity," Humanity 2.0, and the Technium.

In mathematics and physics, a singularity is a point at which the value of a function becomes infinite—for example, in the case of matter that has become infinitely dense at the center of a black hole. The "technological" singularity is an hypothesized future point in history when technological growth becomes uncontrollable and irreversible. Robots and artificial intelligence (AI) are considered the most likely pathways to the technological singularity. For this reason, some observers consider robots and AI existential threats to humanity. These technological "intelligent agents" with their potential capacity for self-reproduction and upgrades could lead to an "intelligence explosion." This combination of intelligence and upgrading could reach a point of rapid expansion and leave humans vulnerable to replacement and even in some scenarios enslavement if not extinction. Some observers believe that we could reach a technological singularity by the middle of this century. Stephen Hawking and Elon Musk are among prominent figures who have identified artificial general intelligence as an existential threat.

The social philosopher Steve Fuller (2012) has argued that we are evolving toward Humanity 2.0, a "singularity" in which we can no longer take the "normal human body" for granted. Humanity 2.0 can be viewed as one of the ways we can address the problems raised by the prospect of a technological singularity. On the one hand, computers, robots, and AI show signs of surpassing the human condition; on the other hand, they are tools—prosthetics—for extending our species specific survival mechanisms. Of course the end result in both cases could be a technological singularity. Computers, robots, and AI may surpass us, or we might become indistinguishable from our prosthetics. Various degrees of flesh-machine integrations can be imagined with different consequences for humanity.

The worry here is an old one: the worry that technology can take on a life of its own. This can be thought of as the Frankenstein problem (Winner, 1977: 7–8). We lack "bearings" in this encounter. The degree, speed, and complexity of technological growth have confounded our abilities to argue, reach conclusions, and make choices. We can no longer trust that our patterns of perceiving and thinking are reliable. Technological realities are outrunning our abilities to make them intelligible. One reaction to this situation is Kevin Kelly's (2012) introduction of the concept of the "Technium," encompassing all of our technologies, machine processes, societies and cultures, and sciences, arts, and humanities in one global system. The sheer complexity of the system gives it increasing autonomy. It evolves and develops its own structures and dynamics. Technologies as small as drones and as large as electrical grids can indeed already become independent of human control. For a hopeful vision of our ability—individually and collectively—to safely navigate the existential threats we face from the basic elements of earth, air, water, and fire, see Peter Denton's (2022) *The End of Technology*.

There is a dark side to our evolutionary story. Species come with an expiration date and 99.9 percent of all the species that E has tinkered into existence are extinct. Besides being a biological species, we humans are a cultural species and that has given us survival advantages. But at the same time culture seems to be the most efficient way to destroy a planetary ecology. Many learned observers, citing things like climate change, the destruction of ecological niches, and dangers to bees, frogs, and butterflies, are persuaded that we are in our last days as a biological species and that the planet's life-giving qualities are themselves in danger. Something like a Technium kingdom may be the only thing that can survive a catastrophic singularity. The Technium may be just another tinkering experiment by E that may extinguish itself in an evolutionary cul de sac or become a new feature of the evolutionary stage, settling in as a seventh kingdom, Technium, alongside the six biological kingdoms: Archaebacteria, Eubacteria, Fungi, Protista, Plants, and Animals.

CONCLUSION

In chapters 1 and 2, I introduced myself as a sociologist of the brain and some of the ingredients of the social network that defines who and what I am as a social being. This was a sociology of the author and a first take on what it means to think sociologically. In this chapter, I have sketched the invention of "the social" as a key feature of the evolutionary process. You now have some of the basic tools, images, and maps you need to navigate the landscape of the brain as a sociological explorer. There is one more critical step. Evolution invented the social; humans had to discover the social. This process is documented in Collins and Makowsky (2010) and Restivo (2018). The discovery of the social evolved from philosophical speculations in the ancient world and crystallized in the nineteenth century in the works of Durkheim, Marx, Weber, Martineau, and others. Sociology, anthropology, and social psychology developed in this period, beginning in the 1840s.

In chapter 4, I will advance our study of the individual in/versus society by considering convergences and divergences in the works of Nietzsche and Marx. In the following two chapters I will explore the implications of the radically social nature of our species at the nexus of our social, cultural, and neurological lives. I will do this by guiding us on a tour of the social body and then we will follow the travels of Einstein's brain.

Chapter 4

Individual and Society

THE "I" AS A GRAMMATICAL ILLUSION

There are many pathways available to the sociologist who wants to look into the contested relationship between the very idea of the "individual" and the very idea of "Society." Does Society program the individual? Can the individual escape the social world that seems to embrace him or her at every turn and in every moment? Is free will possible once we understand the nature and power of Society? I have chosen to explore this contested relationship here by interrogating two of the most brilliant students of the human condition, Friedrich Nietzsche and Karl Marx. The rationale for choosing this path is that it could be said that sociology has developed in part as a dialogue with these two intellectual giants and in part as observations of their own virtual dialogue.

What did Nietzsche mean by alluding to the "I" as a grammatical illusion? In the past I have read sociology into this statement which summarizes a theme that runs throughout Nietzsche's writings: his denial of the reality of the "I." The sociological reading of this denial is based on the widespread belief in the myth of the individual (Callero, 2013) and adherence to the cult of individualism (Barlow, 2013). Nietzsche can't be interviewed, and when we interrogate his writings we are confronted by a brilliant light of all-encompassing inquiry that goes in all directions and doubles and triples back on itself. Weaving our way through this maze cannot lead to definitive conclusions about what Nietzsche meant and what he thought. There are a number of contradictory pathways we have to navigate that nonetheless leave me with some confidence that a sociological reading of Nietzsche's view of the "I" is not idiosyncratic. On Nietzsche's denial of the reality of the "I" see Gardner (2009: 21). A sociological reading of Nietzsche is not clearly reflected in his work. In fact, his work is a coherent chaos situated at the intersection of historical intellectual categories in conflict and "seeking" a resolution, a unification.

Nietzsche's ideas were fueling and being fueled by categories in conflict associated with the emergence of the social sciences in the nineteenth century: transcendentalism/naturalism, the individual/society, and for Nietzsche in particular, great and mediocre humans/the herd, individualism/communitarianism, the practical/the theoretical, and radical skepticism/naturalistic objectivity. There is also a tension in Nietzsche between the sociological imagination and an anti-sociological stance. I will discuss this tension in the last part of this chapter. The overarching tension in this dynamic of opposites is the duality of the Apollonian and the Dionysian. Apollo represents harmony, progress, clarity, logic, and the principle of individuation, whereas Dionysus represents disorder, intoxication, emotion, ecstasy, and unity; the principle of individuation is omitted. We should not be surprised when we encounter difficulties in trying to weave together the ideas of nineteenth-century thinkers into unified, coherent syntheses. From our contemporary standpoint we can see how some unities are beginning to reveal themselves, how the seeds of new theories are being planted.

The practical "I" in Nietzsche is the "I" in "I will . . . " The theoretical "I" is "a mnemonic token, an abbreviating formula" (Gardner, 2009: 9; and see Gemes and May, 2009). This "I will" evokes a Kantian "I think," leading to, respectively, "therefore I do" and "therefore I am." In contemporary sociological terms, these terms are reversed: "I am, therefore I think" and "I do, therefore I am." The problem of inconsistency in Nietzsche's denial of the "I" has been identified by Gardner (2009: 9). A conception of the "I" is indispensable if the individual is to be a value-bearing entity. Nietzsche's philosophy, Gardner continues, is about forging self-affirming individuals (and see West, 2017). We are obliged to assign a reality to the "I" of this value-bearing individual. The problem, to put it differently, is that Nietzsche's self is on the one hand a Platonic fiction (Gardner, 2009: 5) and at the same time fictive in another way "due to its role in masking the real underlying manifold and in the moralization of humanity's self-conception." Nietzsche wrote, Gardner notes, that our concept of unity, of thing, flows from our "I," "our oldest article of faith." The "soul-superstition" is the basis of our oldest realism, "the basis on which we make everything *be* or understand it to *be*, and abandoning it would mean no longer being able to think" (Nietzsche, in Gardner, 2009: 5).

Gardner (2009: 4) writes that the fictional "I" is important for Nietzsche in terms of agency "and the distinction which it implies of doer from deed he regards as a case of motivated error, of taking the same event twice over, once as cause (doer substratum) and once as effect (thing done), all in the service of the slavish fiction of the free will" (Nietzsche, 1887/1994, I 13: 29). That selfhood is an illusion follows from Nietzsche's view of consciousness as epiphenomenal (Gardner, 2009: 3): if consciousness is epiphenomenal, the "I" must be epiphenomenal. But epiphenomena are not fictions, and Nietzsche's thesis is not just that there is an *illusory dimension* to our awareness of the self—that we have false beliefs *about* it—but that its very *existence* is a non-accidental illusion. This is all very confusing even for learned philosophers. But one sees in passages such as aphorism 17 in *Beyond Good and Evil* (Nietzsche, 1886/1989: 24) adumbrations of Ryle's (1949) claim that the mind is nothing but the body at work. One of Nietzsche's most famous remarks is: "the doer is merely a fiction added to the deed" (1887/1994, I: para. 13).

The sociological interpretation of Nietzsche's conception of the "I" as a grammatical illusion has to contend with an essentially psychological concept of the individual as a complex system of competing drives, a dynamic interplay of opposites (Nietzsche,1878/1996: para. 57, 42). After all, he called himself the first psychologist (Nietzsche, 1888/1992: para. 6, 101). What can we say about Nietzsche and sociology?

First, it should be noted that Nietzsche lived in a period I have designated as "The Age of the Social" (1840–1930; Restivo, 2018). The idea of society sui generis was crystallizing during the last half of the nineteenth century in conjunction with the consequences of the earlier voyages of discovery and the birth of anthropology. The intellectual atmosphere of the 1800s was awash in non-European ideas, values, and beliefs. The German universities were reconstructing the history of Christianity. Nietzsche's philosophy is in part a reflection of these movements and an opposition to them. Nietzsche was particularly opposed to the sociological Copernican revolution that put the group at the center of the human universe.

Like Marx, he could dismiss the sociology being sculpted by Comte and Spencer and at the same time show a dawning understanding of "the social" as a part of the natural order. There is no question of Nietzsche's *influence* on sociology. Collins and Makowsky (2010: 60–73) identify Nietzsche as a social theorist and one of the discoverers of "society." In their final assessment, Collins and Makowsky (2010: 73) write that Nietzsche's antagonism to women was paired with a pattern of inquiry that helped to crack the "façade of sentimental idealization and morality . . . [and] reveal the underlying system of domination."

Aspers (2007: 475; *cf.* Karzai, 2019, and his critic Thorpe, 2020) goes further and credits Nietzsche with adopting social constructionist theories. He relies on the classic understanding of social construction introduced by Berger and Luckmann (1966/1991). His discussion focuses on the emergence of meanings in social interaction, the sedimentation of meanings, and their institutionalization. The stronger understanding of social construction I argue for is that the only way humans have of inventing or discovering is by way of their interactions with others in social contexts in the natural ecologies of the Earth and its extra-terrestrial extensions. This sense of social construction depends on the idea that humans come onto the evolutionary stage always, already, and everywhere social. This is alien to Nietzsche's concept of the individual and the herd. Nietzsche's overarching belief is that the group suppresses individuals and destroys their potential for self-creation. The state is to be opposed because it constrains the individual. Take note: it is the state that constrains the individual, not Society, not community.

Sociology on the one hand threatens the freedom of the individual and on the other hand has contributed to demystifying the social. Nietzsche's view of the individual's freedom is one of the illusions that eludes his critical faculties. Even here we must acknowledge his understanding of the social foundations of the individual. Nietzsche's project then becomes to discover a mechanism that would essentially free the individual from these constraints and give birth to the *Übermensch* (variously translated as "Beyond-Man," "Superman," "Overman," "Uberman," or "Superhuman"). Nietzsche's character Zarathustra posits the *Übermensch* as a goal for humanity that represents a shift from otherworldly Christian values. If we dismiss the exaggerated idea that the "Overman" is freed from all social forces and causes, the idea shows a kinship with self-actualization theory.

If we view the Overman as a self-actualized individual, we could argue that Marx too had an Overman agenda. He too wanted a society that allowed individuals to cultivate their gifts and exercise personal freedom. Unlike Nietzsche, an arch-individualist by contrast, Marx (Marx and Engels, 1932/2004: 83) specifically recognized that these goals could only be realized in commune with others. Personal freedom is only possible in the community. While Nietzsche's harsh views of the "herd" blind him to Marx's understanding of the evolutionary significance of the community, one can appreciate that Nietzsche's view of the herd is epitomized in collective actions such as the rallies at Nuremberg. Community is one thing; the dangerous potentials in collective actions and mobs on account of collective effervescence cannot be ignored.

The sociological Nietzsche comes through in his view of science and religion as human made, his analysis of the social origins of values (through ressentiment and in the economic and legal arenas), his concept of the will to power as a theory of social change, and his sociology of power and authority (explicated in his analysis of the evolution of the idea of God and the power of the priesthood).

Nietzsche Meets Marx on the
Battlefield of Self and Society

Some readers will find it curious that I find Nietzsche compatible with anarchism and Marxism (see Thomas, 1985, and Karatani, 2003). The compatibility arises from the elevation of the individual to a value in itself and the resistance to the state. The difference lies in the stronger sociological understanding of the individual as through and through social in anarchism and Marxism, as opposed to Nietzsche's "Overman."

At first sight, Nietzsche and Marx couldn't be more different. They championed, respectively, passion versus reason, the individual versus the collective, hierarchy versus equality, the Overman versus the masses and the oppressed. This seems correct in terms of the big canvas that portrays them. However, no one defended reason with more intensity than Nietzsche (1881/2007: para. 18, 26–27): "Nothing has been more dearly bought than the minute portion of human reason and feeling of liberty upon which we now pride ourselves." And he writes about the importance of making our "experiences a matter of conscience for knowledge" (Nietzsche, 1887/1974: para. 319, 253). We are urged to interrogate what we really experienced: what was the context of the experience, was our reason bright, our will opposed to self-deception and "bold in resisting the fantastic"? He rails against those, especially the religious, who "thirst after things that go *against reason*," making them more susceptible to "miracles" and "rebirths" and "the voices of little angels!" Those of us who thirst after reason are ready to make ourselves scientific experiments constantly scrutinizing our experiences: "We ourselves wish to be our experiments and guinea pigs." Who among us has the capacity and courage to carry out such experiments? There is a reason Nietzsches are rare!

Marx, the scientific socialist, understood better than anyone of his era that science was social relations, indeed that scientists themselves were social relations. Modern bourgeois science as a social institution was a product and an ingredient of modern capitalist society. Marx (1956: 110–11; 1973: 699ff) introduced the idea of an alternative "human science" that he associated with a new social order. Science-as-it-is would be negated, and a new science—dealienated, integrated but not unified, holistic, and global—would emerge.

Marx and Nietzsche agreed in important ways about religion and the state. Nietzsche understood that religion can give people a feeling of control over what they often experience as the chaos of life, powerlessness in the face of suffering, and the meaning of life being always out of reach. Religion can also give some people power over others and maximize the religious ones' prosperity. Marx, famous for the slogan "religion is the opiate [sometimes given as 'opium'] of the people," leads up to that by writing that "religion is the sigh of the oppressed creature, the heart of a heartless world, just as it is the spirit of a spiritless situation" (Marx, 1847/1957: 42). Marx and Nietzsche understand religion as a social and cultural phenomenon. It is not a gateway to or a revelation of a transcendental or supernatural reality. Both discuss the power dimension of religion in society. Marx sees this in terms of the empowerment of those in search of meaning and basic survival under the oppressive conditions of capitalism, but he does not rely on Nietzsche's idea of a universal will to power. In brief, Marx's approach is social, political, and economic; Nietzsche's approach blends classical philosophy and contemporary psychology.

We can see an important commonality if we notice Marx's critique of capitalism and his vision of a future society governed "from each according to his ability to each according to his need," and Nietzsche's critique of Christianity and his recognition of the need for a new system of values that would guide meaningful lives for humanity. Here a powerful debate awaits us about whether there is a way to bridge Marx's struggle for equality and Nietzsche's view of the doctrine of equality as a "venomous poison."

Rhetoric matters. There is no question that Nietzsche's militarist perspective and a rhetoric of "degenerates," "masters" and "slaves," and the "weak" encouraged racists and war-mongers to speak in his name on behalf of beliefs and actions that would have repulsed him. It is important to acknowledge the role of his sister Elizabeth and her fascist husband Bernhard Förster in promoting this reading of Nietzsche. Similarly, Marx would have been repulsed by Stalinism and modern so-called communist societies.

In general, their differences are minimized once we recognize that they were both opposed to state power and champions of what today we would call self-actualization. This gives both Marx and Nietzsche anarchist credentials in spite of their antipathy to the anarchism of their time. Perhaps their differences all stem from the difference between the concept of "will to power" (Nietzsche) and "class conflict" (Marx). This difference underlies their critique of contemporary philosophy. Marx's critique is based on the fact that philosophy in the West grows out of capitalism. Nietzsche's critique stems from philosophy as a product of the will to power. Nietzsche (1889, 1895/1968: para. 34, 86–87) views the anarchist as "the mouthpiece of the *declining* strata of society, righteously demanding rights, justice, and equality." The anarchist, Nietzsche argues, lacks culture and needs to find someone to blame for his suffering, his vile feelings. Nietzsche viewed anarchism as a system of complaints arising from weakness. The anarchist and the Christian share a need to blame someone for one's suffering, and both seek revenge.

It is easy to conclude that Nietzsche's arch-individualism, culminating in the "Overman," and his resistance to the "herd" overwhelm the clear sociological voices in his philosophy. He seems to say yes to the individual and no to the community. The situation is unfolded in an intriguing series of essays collected by Julian Young (2015). Young situates Nietzsche's philosophy in a German tradition of religious or quasi-religious communitarianism (Young, 2015: 2). How, then, does the demand for community cohere with the significance Nietzsche attaches to the exceptional individual? That individual (recall Hegel's "world historical individual") is the agent of change who understands how the community's ethos needs to evolve to adapt to an environment in flux.

CONCLUSION

The modern state has declined into an agonistic arena of selfish interests (nihilism). Parallel to Plato arguing for installing philosopher kings to establish a functioning "republic" and Comte's proposal for a human community ruled by sociology priests, Nietzsche argues for a society ruled by artist-kings. His Zarathustra gives us a community that is not for everyman but for a "diachronic elite of geniuses," a spiritual community dedicated to perfecting humanity without the loss of individuality. Young's book lays out the basic features of Nietzsche's inner debate about individual and community and how that inner debate has been assessed by philosophers of Nietzschean philosophy.

The birth of sociology in the nineteenth century brought with it the beginnings of the conflict between psychology and sociology over the issue of the individual versus society. Marx and Nietzsche share many of the same sensitivities to the societal and cultural transformations working their way through their century. At the end of the day, Nietzsche was going to rely on the exceptional individual to bring us through the crisis; Marx relegated that task to the working class. Looking at Nietzsche and Marx through the lens of contemporary sociology it is clear that Marx was the more sophisticated sociological thinker. He valued the individual as much as Nietzsche did but understood the individual as through and through social.

Chapter 5

The Social Body in Society and Politics

A Nietzschean Overture
(1) There is only body, a first approximation; (2) Consciousness is a network of communication; (3) "O those Greeks! They knew how to live. What is required for that is to stop courageously at the surface, the fold, the skin, to adore appearance, to believe in forms, tones, words, the whole Olympus of appearance. Those Greeks were superficial—*out of profundity*
(Nietzsche, 1887: xii; my translation).

LONELINESS, THE INDIVIDUAL, AND SOCIETY

If the late twentieth century was in one dimension the Age of the Body, the twenty-first century has challenged our understanding of the body imperative by exposing us to two pandemics: COVID-19 and POTUS-45, the Trump presidency. COVID-19 forced us to confront the social nature of the body. For the most part studies of the body in the late twentieth century focused on the influences and contexts of technology, biology, and medicine on bodies. COVID-19 forced us to return to sociological imperatives in body studies. POTUS-45, the presidency of Donald Trump, forced us to consider how threats to democracy were threats to the body as a center of freedom and liberation. We have seen one of the consequences of this threat dramatically realized in the Supreme Court's ruling, announced while I was editing this manuscript, overturning *Roe v. Wade*. The ruling came with barely hidden agendas that threaten same-sex marriage and access to contraception.

The seventeenth-century philosopher Blaise Pascal (1995/1670: 37, DIVERSION 136) remarked that all of our problems stem from our inability to sit quietly alone in a room. Kings and peasants alike, without wars and struggles for survival to divert them, men and women without games and circuses to distract them, cannot find consolation when they are alone and start to think about the threats they face, the challenges of everyday life they deal with, and the finality of death.

Many studies have demonstrated that humans become uncomfortable when forced to sit in an empty room with only their own thoughts to dwell on. Social science offers an answer to this problem that social psychologist Steve Taylor (2012) has diagnosed as "humania." It follows from the fact that we are culturally victims of the myth and cult of the individual. We experience ourselves as individual, isolated beings. Left to our own devices, we become locked in a spiral of increasing awareness of loneliness. One factor is that we have been loosened from our deeply social natures by cultural developments, especially in the industrial West and its geopolitical satellites. In evolutionary perspective, we humans arrive on the evolutionary stage already, always, and everywhere social. We do not arrive as individuals who then become social by way of some "social contract" event. We arrive social, and culture individuates us (Restivo, 2018: 104–7). Another factor is the volume of our cultural capital (see further on).

Loosening us from our evolutionary social nature produces what I've designated "dissocism." This is a spectrum of alienative conditions that blind us to our social nature and make it impossible for us to "see" the social and to see it as the causal foundation of all of our thoughts, emotions, and behaviors. Contrast this with the reigning neuroist (Brothers, 2001: 3) assumption that our brains are the source of all of our thoughts, emotions, and behaviors. This is reflected in the rationales for the various late twentieth- and early twenty-first century international brain initiatives, including Bush in 1990 and Obama in 2013. Under these conditions the social problem of loneliness is exacerbated. COVID-19 has underlined and brought to light the nature and implications of neglecting our social nature. It has alerted those of us prepared to see its implications to the fallacy of the transparency of introspection. Our experience of our selves as free-willing agents is as much an illusion as our experience that the Earth does not move (see chapter 3).

Loneliness has been a concern for many observers of the human condition, especially in America, for some time now. Social isolation or rejection disrupts our thinking, our will power, and our immune systems (Cacioppo and Patrick, 2008). It is for this reason that solitary confinement should be considered "cruel and unusual punishment." Loneliness in the context of modern industrial technological societies—lack of connections—may be the key to violent behaviors ranging from bullying to street violence and school shootings. It's not too much of a leap to suggest that it might play a role in terrorism and warfare. Not only should we not underestimate the relevance of the loss of community in explaining violence, we should also pay more attention to the relevance of touching in a radically social species. Fear of and barriers to touching (and sex, which is a complicated extrapolation of touching) are implicated along with loneliness in many if not most of the problems of the human condition (Montagu, 1971). We misunderstand and vastly underestimate the significance and power of sex, which is everywhere. My undergraduate mentor, anthropologist Burt Aginsky, described it as a force of nature like gravity and labeled that force "sexity." Our failures in this arena are a breeding ground for confusion, frustration, and violent behaviors.

Loneliness is not just an individual phenomenon. The separation of groups and cultures may cause a kind of collective loneliness. Ecumenical thinkers like Karen Armstrong (Charter for Compassion) and the Dalai Lama have argued that world peace could be based on the compassion that is at the center of all religious traditions. The problem is that compassion is a centripetal force and reinforces the boundaries that separate groups and cultures. This force tends to overwhelm any centrifugal forces that might help to link us across our cultural differences. There are certainly cases in which the centrifugal forces of compassion can be mobilized to support communication and exchange across national borders and across barriers of sex, gender, race, class, and ethnicity. But the differences represented in all these categories of our lives are intensified by the centripetal force of compassion. And this breeds acts of physical and emotional violence across these categories.

Social ties do not necessarily mean that loneliness and its negative effects have been overcome. Consider the cases of gangs and cults. People in gangs and cults have social ties, but these groups are associated with individual psychiatric morbidity. Social ties have to be considered in their cultural contexts to determine their impact on loneliness (Harper et al., 2008; Macfarlane, 2019). Okruszek et al. (2021) offer evidence that objective isolation is associated with social cognitive abilities, but that is not the case for perceived loneliness. They acknowledge the research that demonstrates loneliness has a higher impact on mortality rates than hypertension or obesity. Loneliness can be linked to objective social isolation, but loneliness does not imply social isolation. A marriage, for example, may be perceived as loving and caring and be objectively detached and lacking in affection.

We radically social humans have become increasingly disconnected from each other. The resulting loneliness many of us have been exposed to has damaged our individual and collective health. In *Bowling Alone*, Putnam (2000) documents the ways in which we have become increasingly disconnected from each other. Putnam may indeed have deftly diagnosed the damage that loneliness has done to our individual and collective health, but this kind of analysis is not new. It became visible as part of the collateral social damage of the industrial revolution. It is iconically represented in the distinction between Gemeinschaft (communal society) and Gesellschaft (associational society), discussed in chapter 3. There was a sense of loss—a loss of community, a loss of connection—in these dichotomies, not a sense of progress. It is time we gave serious attention to the evolutionary sociology lesson that humans arrive on the evolutionary stage already, everywhere, and always social. This leads to new ways of thinking about body, self, brain, mind, and consciousness. And it gives us a new way to understand creative thinking and genius. There are no "lone wolf" geniuses. Even when alone or in isolation the person is a social being.

Rhythm and the Social Order

Let's go back to the nature of the body in this social context. The following theory builds on the works of Collins (2004), Bassetti and Bottazzi (2015), Farrera and Ramos-Fernández (2022), Goffman (1982), Keller, Novembre, and Hove (2014), and Warner (1988); and see the section on "the field concept" and the rationale for introducing it in chapter 10. When humans come into contact with other humans a field is generated that engages a process of rhythmic entrainment. This field carries emotional communication and consciousness. Human bodies are rhythmic systems, essentially vibrating entities. Our postural vibrations are constantly adjusting to what comes under our gaze, whether an object like a painting or plants, animals, objects, and other humans. Dance is the coarse-level expression of the fine-grained rhythmicity that is innate to all levels of life from cells to bodies; and even social systems have their rhythms, even societies and groups dance.

Consciousness originates in the social world (Cohen and Rapport, 1995; Whitehead, 2008) as a by-product of the innate rhythmicity of humans. It is our capacity for dance as an "in-between" conduit that generates consciousness. In evolutionary terms we are musical first (Mithen, 2005). Or perhaps musicality, proto-language, and dance are all part of the same evolutionary moment. Humans have "evolved with nervous systems that pay attention to each other: there is always the possibility of fighting, or spreading an alarm; or, on the positive side, possible sexual contact and more generally sociable gestures" (Collins, 2004: 54). In a footnote (380n4), Collins refers to Turner's (2002) use of evidence from paleontology and cladistics, primate behavior, and brain physiology to draw attention to the conditions that led to humans developing elaborate emotional repertoires. These provided the scaffolding for the capacity in humans for social coordination, a capacity first observed in the non-human primates and carried to new levels among humans.

My thesis is that bodily co-presence induces rhythmic entrainment (RE). It does not require that people "do anything." Classically, for example, Collins (2004: 52) gives the example of peoples' activities in the hours leading up to midnight on New Year's Eve, especially the activity of making noises at each other and together. This and other group activities "lead" to entrainment. By contrast, I contend that these activities enhance a base-level RE that is engendered as soon as human bodies come into proximity. I don't know of any way to measure this base level or at what distance it kicks in, but it's probably optimal at face-to-face conversational distances. We should expect different forms and levels of RE when certain aspects of the body/brain system are impaired or missing. Not being able to hear or see or missing one or more limbs will alter individual rhythms, and REs in such cases will differ from REs between people with all senses and bodily integrity intact. REs are also impacted by culture, class, ethnicity, sex, and gender. REs are the fuel of collective effervescence (defined below).

Entrainment is a basic concept in biomusicology. It refers to synchronization to an external rhythm (e.g., tapping, drumming, music, dancing). It has also been studied in dance, communication, and motor coordination. One theory holds that entrainment evolved in humans as a way to achieve "battle trance" (Jordania, 2011). More generally, the enhancement of collective identity had survival value in battle where it helps humans lose their individuality. This exaggerates the extent to which individual awareness had evolved in our earliest ancestors. However, generalized warfare does not appear before about 6000 BCE, by which time a high enough level of individuality had been developed to perhaps necessitate "battle trance."

A general theory of entrainment treats RE in humans as a basic feature of life that allows organisms to perceive and respond to rhythmic stimuli. Social entrainment arises on the scaffolding of spatiotemporal coordination. I haven't found any indication that students of RE outside of sociology have linked it to consciousness (see, however, Mithen, 2005). For a general theory of entrainment, see Phillips-Silver, Aktipis, and Bryant (2010). These authors speculate that social entrainment may facilitate higher-level organization that requires real-time information sharing between or among individuals that are producing and/or processing rhythmic information. In complex systems with highly interdependent components, the ability to transmit information quickly and effectively can promote efficiency at a higher level and even enable otherwise impossible functionality. In a variety of species, coordinated activities may play a role in promoting higher-level functions. This hints obliquely at the possibility that RE is the source of mind, consciousness and emotions, but these authors do not include this possibility in their theory. They also depend on an individualistic physical model for generating entrainment rather than the natural mutual presence model I argue for.

RE chains lead to collective effervescence (CE), first identified by Durkheim. It is usually used to refer at the group level. When a group comes together and participates in the same activity at an event, RE creates a collective experience under a relatively unified focus of attention, producing the same or similar emotions and consciousness. But CE emerges at all levels, from dyads and triads to large audiences, gatherings, and ceremonies. CE also arises at the level of the individual under circumstances of inward focus and attention.

If you do not have access to this social model and you are restricted to brain-centric thinking, you might solve the hard problem of consciousness by proposing a transducer theory. This is exactly what Robert Epstein (2021) has done. Epstein, a neuroscientist, begins by identifying certain mysteries that require explanation. Epstein's mysteries include spirits, dreams, and the immaterial realms transcending the reality we know. We have had a sociological theory that explains these phenomena since the late 1800s in the work of Emile Durkheim. Once we understand rituals, emotions, and collective effervescence we have the basic ingredients for explaining the origin of religious experience and the gods. This forms the foundation for a general rejection of transcendence. The explanation of Epstein's other mysteries then fall readily into place. Epstein's transducer theory is a mechanical solution, but it assumes a brain that doesn't exist, an isolated biological brain that operates independently of its cultural environment. Thinking in terms of social selves, social bodies, and social brains stays within the framework of cultural phenomena and doesn't require an electro-mechanical solution. Nonetheless, perhaps what we have here are two sides of the same coin. We have a phenomenon which lends itself to two different theories depending on whether the approach is brain centered or social centered. The two solutions are mirror images of each other. And since the electro-mechanical biological brain is still a reality in the social brain model, Epstein's model, like other neurotechnologies, may have therapeutic and analytical applications.

There is an historical context for the rhythm theory I have just outlined. The idea has a kinship with theories variously labeled resonance, synchrony, coherence, and shared vibrations. The general theory of resonance is a prominent part of neuroscientific, physical, biological, and philosophical efforts to explain consciousness (Bandyopadhyay, 2019; Crick and Koch, 1990; Dehaene, 2014; Fries, 2005, 2015; Freeman and Vitello, 2006; Grossberg, 2017; Koch, 2004; Pocket, 2000, 2012; Sahu et al., 2013, 2013; and Singh et al., 2018). The general theory of resonance proposed by Hunt and Schooler (2020) builds on these developments. They argue that rhythmicity is universal; everything in the universe is vibrating whether we adopt an up-down or a down-up causal format. But this literature does not generally treat rhythmic entrainment in humans as a specific case of resonance. Hunt and Schooler implicitly include humans in their theory, which holds that mind and matter are two sides of the same coin; consciousness is ubiquitous. This is known as panpsychism, the doctrine or belief that everything material, however small, has an element of individual consciousness. This is more metaphysics than science. There may be a rationale for a theory that some elementary ingredients of consciousness are present already at the atomic level in the same way that the potential for life is present. This does not mean that atoms are either alive or conscious in any meaningful substantive way. Panpsychism undermines itself by introducing an element of spiritualism into resonance theory. However, there is a great deal of theory that offers a rationale for my approach to rhythmic entrainment in humans as the basis for consciousness. This requires a synthesis of Durkheim's sociology and Collins's work on emotions with the literature on resonance and rhythmicity discussed in this chapter.

Socialness is a fuel and our social being must be constantly refueled. The amount of fuel in our "self-tank" is measured in units of cultural capital. I adapt the term introduced by Bourdieu and Passeron (1977/1990; and see Bourdieu, 1985). I use the term "cultural capital" to refer specifically to the forms of cultural capital that can be embodied. That is, what kinds and parts of accumulated cultural knowledge can be held in a memory cache (self-tank) with sufficient stability and sustainability to fuel one's conscious awareness of and access to the cache? Language is a primary example of this form of cultural capital. The larger the tank and the more cultural capital it holds at any given time establish the limits of sanity when alone or in isolation.

Loneliness is a social disease and can kill you or disable you in various ways and to different degrees. The Pascal problem of being alone arises in part because of our innate radically social nature but also because and to the extent that we go into the room alone with a fuel tank almost empty of cultural capital. The more cultural capital in our tank the easier it is to be alone, within limits (Restivo, 2018: 81–83). Some recent research (Chang et al., 2022; Masterson, 2022) suggests that the negative effects of loneliness can be offset by engaging in meaningful activities. The active use of skills and concentration work better than passive activities like watching television. Being engrossed in what you are doing puts you in a flow state. Watching television doesn't engage your skills and concentration in this way. The concept of "flow" drawn on in this research is based on Csikszentmihalyi (2008, 2014).

These efforts are grounded in a critique of the traditional understanding of science and ultimately of the Western subject as universal norms. To approach this in terms of an orientalist/occidentalist or nordist/australist perspective connects the theory and critique of science to "the secular notion of an individual 'I' as an abstract and universal consciousness free of all embodiment and locality" (Yegenoglu, 1998; on the north/south divide, see Diamond, 1998; Richards and Ruivenkamp, 1996; Seabrook, 1993; Strathern, 1992; and see Restivo and Loughlin, 2000). The Western subject (already gendered to subordinate the female and the feminine, as well as raced and classed) is brought into being as a universal norm in the process of the West's expansion.

The historian W. H. McNeill (1963: 569) described this in terms of three talismans of power: (1) a deep-rooted pugnacity and recklessness operating by means of (2) a complex military technology, most notably in naval matters; and (3) a population inured to a variety of diseases which had long been endemic throughout the Old World ecumene. Note especially the references to pugnacity and recklessness.

The "universal subject" norm denies the subject's dependence on the Other and produces the illusion of autonomy and freedom. In fact, this abstract and universal *consciousness* was always embodied, male, and European, whether indigenous or transplanted. Women and non-European men—even if they achieved the required education—could enter science only as surrogates, disciples, or through passing (that is, by adopting the language, gestures, postures, attitudes, and values of Euro-American men).

The Myth and Cult of the Individual

Consider the very idea of "genius." In John Wayne's America, genius has "Big Shoulders" (the Comanche chief Scar's name for Wayne's character in the 1956 movie *The Searchers*) and little room for women who might want to claim the genius mantle. Gertrude Stein made room for herself by saying out loud, "I am a genius." She went on to domesticate the concept in documenting her relationship with Alice B. Toklas. But Albert Einstein is *America's and the world's* genius of geniuses. In 1916, and not yet forty years old, he predicted gravity waves (a consequence of the General Theory of Relativity). It took one hundred years before scientists had technologies and computers that were a match for Einstein's brain and that could detect gravity waves. When I was a young boy in love with science and math, Einstein was already a scientific saint. And when he died on April 18, 1955, his brain became a sacred scientific relic. Eventually the sliced, preserved pieces of Einstein's brain began a journey across John Wayne's America, from sea to shining sea, and beyond. The search was on for Einstein's genius in the architecture of his brain. This seemed perfectly reasonable in John Wayne's America. When we identify Einstein as a genius, and when we assume the secrets to that genius are in his genes and neurons, we learn more about ourselves and our culture than we do about Einstein.

When Orson Welles was asked to name his three favorite directors he said "John Ford, John Ford, and John Ford." Ford constantly toyed with the relationship between truth and fiction, fact and legend. In *The Man Who Shot Liberty Valence* (1962) Ford created an exit line that belongs in the definition of the American mythos. Maxwell Scott (played by Carleton Young) is ready to publish a story about Senator Ransom Stoddard (James Stewart) and the mythical figure he has become for killing the villain Liberty Valence (Lee

Marvin). In the closing scenes, Scott learns that Stoddard didn't kill Valence. Scott tears up his notes. Stoddard says: "You're not going to use the story, Mr. Scott?" Scott replies, "No, sir. This is the West, sir. When the legend become fact, print the legend."

Valence was actually killed by Tony Doniphon, John Wayne's character. Here Wayne is associated with the conflict between the autonomous hero affirming the myth of individualism and the eternal recurrence of the myth. It seems to get defeated from time to time as collective community interests come into play. Ethan Edwards (Wayne's character in *The Searchers*) embodies the American myth of individualism, the hero who stands outside of society and its surface norms, values, and beliefs. Edwards, like many of our heroes, appears often enough to feed our need for violence, and then disappears to wander across America's spacious skies, amber waves of grain, purple mountain majesties, and fruited plain. He leaves a trail of masculinity, patriotism, self-reliance, and self-responsibility in his wake. Occasionally we may get images of something more than a cowboy riding or walking off into the sunset. There may be a hug, a kiss, a look of longing, a farm saved from disaster, villains dispatched, and a town's solidarity restored, something that has the scent of community. But it doesn't last in John Wayne's America.

Individualism returns again and again. And this is why John Wayne the movie icon is the embodiment of the myth of individualism and even a kind of genius of masculine posture, pride, and stride. He is America's icon of heroic individualism and rugged masculinity among white males but to varying degrees among others who buy into American exceptionalism and the myth of individualism. One doesn't usually associate Einstein with rugged masculinity, but his numerous affairs and his attraction for women speak to some kind of masculinity and certainly something gendered about his genius. It made the role of his wife Mileva virtually invisible in his life and in his work.

John Wayne's America sings the hymns of individualism, of self-interest, of capitalism unleashed. Capitalism, however, is not an actual economy but an ideology (Restivo, 2018: 186–93). Its embodiments reflect its internal contradictions. The classic robber baron, individualist to his core, is also a philanthropist—and this tension is revealed in all of our heroes. Einstein is in this context a transformation of that mythology and its conflict with the mythology of "we the people," *e pluribus unum*. He was, from the public's perspective, unique, individual, living in his own world by his own impenetrable rules—but he was also the great humanitarian. That is why it seemed so natural to imagine that the secret of Einstein's genius could be read from the architecture of his brain, the inner landscape of a unique individual outside of society, culture, history, time, and space. And what a landscape we imagined it might be like. Awe-inspiring, of course, like the landscape of Monument Valley, Utah, in the opening scenes of *The Searchers*.

If individualism is a myth—if, as Nietzsche claimed, the "I" is a grammatical illusion (see chapter 4)—can we say anything about Einstein with confidence that doesn't erase his obvious uniqueness? Developments in neuroscience (especially environmental-enrichment studies and mirror neuron and plasticity research), social neuroscience, epigenetics, social science, and network theory between 1950 and the 1990s do pose challenges to Einstein's uniqueness. They don't erase it, but they do force us to rethink the nature of his uniqueness. With respect to his physics, for example, the idea of mass-energy equivalence was not new; it was already in the conversations of physicists by the 1870s. Henri Poincaré published papers on the relativity theory in 1904 and 1905 (Einstein's *annus mirabilis*).

Uniqueness is not a matter of genes, neurons, quantum phenomena, or the biological brain. Einstein's uniqueness is defined by the uniqueness of the social networks he encountered as his life unfolded. If his brain holds any clues to his creativity, those clues would be functions of how his social and cultural environments impacted the architecture of his brain. This idea is reflected in the social brain model, introduced into the neuroscience literature by Leslie Brothers in 1990. Einstein's dead brain could not be a narrative of innate genius. The story of his genius has to be a story of connections in the world at large.

Genius: The Very Idea

The lone wolf genius only lives in John Wayne's America. The term "genius" rests on the concept of the individual as an entity that stands apart from society, history, and culture. Genius even escapes time and space. The mythical genius is "an island entire of itself," but "he" is not alone. Etymologically, the genius has a guiding spirit, a tutelary deity. This makes the genius not only an island unto himself but a god, and classically masculine. If genius were simply a matter of genes, neurons, or "ineffables," geniuses would appear at random, scattered haphazardly across various disconnected cultural landscapes. But genius clusters. And genius clusters do not appear randomly but during the rapid decline or ascent of civilizations and cultural areas (Kroeber, 1963: 7–27, 838–46; Mercier and Sperber, 2017: 315–27; Simonton, 1999: 199–241; Weiner, 2016). I sketch Einstein's genius cluster in chapter 6. These developments give us a new way to think about consciousness.

Consciousness: The Hard Problem?

The so-called "hard problem" of consciousness is the problem of explaining the relationship between the physical (material, "hard") phenomena of the brain and brain processes on the one hand and mind and consciousness (immaterial, "soft") on the other. Classically, the problem is: How do brains create minds and consciousness? Theologically, the problem revolves around bodies and souls. The very statement of the problem has trapped it in the jurisdiction of philosophers, psychologists, biologists, cognitive scientists, and neuroscientists. Physicists, who believe they can explain anything, and theologians who can explain things that don't exist, are also prominent players in the consciousness game. The "hard problem" is hard because the wrong scientists using the wrong tools have been looking for it in the wrong place. They have been looking for it in the brain and ignoring an idea that has been around since the 1800s, that consciousness is a network of social relationships and communication. But social relationships as the source of causes that impact our behaviors, emotions, and thoughts are invisible in John Wayne's America. They are made invisible by the myth of individualism. This in turn invalidates sociology as a science and as a science that might have the key to the hard problem.

Psychologists and philosophers of brain and mind regularly start to home in on this reality. They might recognize, for example, that we are more sociological entities than single, unified psychological entities. But if they interpret this as a metaphor, as some do (the prominent psychologist Michael Gazzaniga, 1985, for one) they will be diverted to their default biological explanations for consciousness and social institutions like religion. Their failures create an explanatory vacuum physicists are all too enthusiastic to fill with their tool kit of quantum concepts. This is the classic case of the wrong scientists with the wrong tools looking in the wrong place, guided more by what they experience as the introspective transparency of their own minds (an illusion) than by science. Roger Penrose (1989) is a classic example of a physicist guided by his own introspective experience of consciousness and thinking toward a theory of mind. It is not my intention to drive the physical and natural sciences out of the game. However, it is becoming more and more apparent that society and culture are implicated in how the brain works. This is an argument not merely for bringing sociology and anthropology to the table, but perhaps putting them at the head of the table.

Consider that philosophers of mind like John Searle (1992) and neuroscientists like Antonio Damasio (1994) have recognized that social and cultural factors must play a role in cognition and consciousness. Searle says he doesn't know how to mobilize these factors, and Damasio finds trying to bring them to bear in brain studies too daunting. Neither one of these particular players seems to be aware that sociologists exist who do know how to mobilize these factors and do not find this daunting. They certainly know that sociologists exist, so I can only conclude that they are not prepared to take them seriously.

The myth of individualism causes social blindness, the inability to see the social, and then to fail to see it as a causal force shaping our behaviors, thoughts, and emotions. This is dissocism, and there is a dissocism spectrum disorder. To the extent that we are all to varying degrees victims of social blindness, what I've been writing will undoubtedly be counter-intuitive for many readers. The way to make this intuitive is to consider again the difference between our experience that the earth does not move and the reality of its complex movements through space (as we saw in chapter 3).

The studies of Einstein's brain proved in the end to be sterile. They were guided by neuroist assumptions (mind and consciousness are brain phenomena), a dissocist perspective, the fallacy of introspective transparency, and a conspiracy of mythologies: the myth of individualism, the myth of the brain-in-a-vat (think *The Matrix* and speculations that we are a simulation; see chapter 8), and the myth of brain-centric thinking reinforced by gene-centric thinking. In a 2006 study of Einstein's brain, J. A. Colombo and his colleagues found nothing distinctive about the four blocks they'd studied. They saw a diseased brain rather than the brain of a genius. They criticized the earlier studies of Einstein's brain for their inconsistencies and methodological flaws and doubted whether microscopic neuroanatomy studies could ever prove useful.

The "I" is a grammatical illusion. We are all social in a radical sense as opposed to being individuals in a radical sense. From birth to the present, contexts and networks have been shaping my thinking and my "choices." And yours too.

Wait. Isn't it possible that there is some sort of dialectical relationship between the "I" and social structures or networks, some "slippage" between individual and society? Some social scientists do indeed take this path. For those who do, there is always a volatile potential for prioritizing psychology and biology over social science. There is always the danger that their introspective sense of self will override the science of the social. That's why I think it's wise to assume that it's social networks all the way down.

A Little Politics Couldn't Hurt

The main political lesson of the POTUS-45 era in the United States is that our Constitution needs to be updated. We have learned that it cannot protect us as persons or our physical and natural bodies from actions that undermine the rule of law, democracy, and progress toward a more perfect union. It cannot protect us from demagoguery and authoritarianism in the Oval Office itself, never mind in other governmental arenas. The following proposals assume that democracy is a system which should strive for, reinforce, and protect liberty and justice for all. In fact, I find anarchism a more promising and healthier political alternative (Restivo, 2016). For the moment, I will assume democracy. In that case, we should consider several new amendments to reinforce the Constitution's protections of life, liberty, and the pursuit of happiness in a democratic society. It is long past the time for a Constitutional Convention. We are no longer living in 1776 or 1791. What does this have to do with the body? Non-democratic governments must exert harsh discipline over the body. In societal terms, this means that bodies will be sexed, gendered, raced, classed, and enslaved.

We have been witnessing this principle take on a new life in America that has in this century seen the crystallization of a fascist American Taliban with highly visible representatives in the Republican party. A great many of our lawmakers are averse to a politics of compassion and are enemies of science, education, and the life of the mind. This is true everywhere, but America is the model for the politics of enslavement veiled in democratic slogans. Too many of our lawmakers believe the individual should bear the burdens of social structural outcomes that interfere with the quality of life. The absurdity of using the Dow Jones average as the main public indicator of the health of an economy marked by intolerable levels of poverty and unconscionable gaps in wealth and income should finally be recognized. The lack of a politics of compassion means that health care, social security, and other parts of the social safety net are always going to be at risk. We may need to test the capacity of the law to institute compassion in the short run and hope that, in the long run, compassion will become a norm of our culture. We have seen such an achievement in practical (not utopian) terms in other nations.

I noted earlier that unadulterated compassion is a centripetal force that reinforces boundaries and restricts connections across social categories, groups, cultures, and nations. Are there compassionate politicians in America? Of course there are. But most cannot see beyond capitalism and democracy as friends of economic and political progress and not of the people. The ultimate politics of the body requires that we recognize that capitalism is not, has never been, and can never be an actual economic system. It is rather an ideological smoke screen that masks a system of exploitation. If an ideology's basic assumptions violate the laws of nature and the human condition, any effort at any level to implement the ideology will be destructive. Such violations in capitalist models, for example, include rational self-interest, the invisible hand, the "free market," an even playing field for buyers and sellers, a profits-first philosophy prior to or without accounting for people and environments, a homogeneous plane assumption (equal distribution of resources—quality and quantity—across the planet), and competition. The reality is that the planet and its flora, fauna, ecologies, humans, and societies are character-ized by inequalities. Furthermore, as Darwin already recognized, ecologies and environments thrive on cooperative principles more than on competitive ones. Any viable economic system has to be based on these inequalities and the cooperative principle (Montagu,1952). No model that deserves the label "capitalism" does this. No actual economy has ever manifested the collec-tion of features in any model of capitalism. Capitalism is an ideology, not an actual working economy. The standard features that define any of the models of capitalism fail to conform with the social, cultural, environmental, and planetary ecological realities of the Earth and its peoples. Any effort to put an economy into operation based on a capitalist model will almost immediately have to import non-capitalist features (handicapping) to avoid environmental and sociocultural disasters. Following such an ideology full-tilt will destroy ecological and human systems. Even Adam Smith (1759/2021) handicapped "capitalism" in his theory of moral sentiments, which is ignored by capitalists and almost everyone else.

Democracy is only valuable as a stepping stone to anarchy. I do not speak of anarchy here as a term that connotes chaos and disorder but rather of anar-chism understood as one of the social sciences (Kropotkin, 1908). Translated onto the political arena, it gives a government that is decentralized to such an extent that we humans become self-governing. We become the caretakers of the planet, of our communities, and of our bodies.

Interlude—Once More, Science

A word finally on how science fits into this perspective. I've noted that all knowledge claims escape their evidence and must be considered highly pre-sumptive, corrigible, and fallible. There is no justification for investing any scientific claim with positive or absolute belief; everything is in flux and subject to criticism and change. That doesn't leave us entirely groundless. Grounding our sciences in our experience of crossing the street, an imperative of pursuing the profundity of the surface, modifies the idea that everything is in flux. The profundity of the surface is not the end of inquiry but a portal to deeper and even more profound levels and dimensions of knowledge. But we must begin with this. We should not invest scientific claims with absolute belief. This helps us limit ungrounded deterministic, universal, and invariant claims. It does not eliminate them. The reason is that without certain levels of closure in the systems of our everyday lives, life would be impossible.

Our world gives us levels of closure that make social life possible and subject to definitive descriptions in practice. I have made an effort to pre-serve "sciences," the basic human capacity for reason. Nothing has cost us so dearly, Nietzsche (1881/2007: 26) wrote, as that "little bit of reason and sense of freedom . . . which now constitutes our pride." There is a caveat that modifies the fact that facts of the matter are presumptive. The caveat is rooted in the recalcitrance of everyday reality's factual closures that make life possible. Anything goes, but even anarchists leave buildings through front doors and not by leaping out of windows. And those factual closures are what make a practical explanatory causal science possible.

Imagine an alternative to my book *Society and the Death of God* (2021) titled *Society and the Death of the Flat Earth*. After reviewing all the available evidence through the centuries, should we be prepared to argue to "near certainty" or "absolute certainty" that the Earth is not flat? We cannot be concerned about or fearful of alienating people any more than Galileo was in defending heliocentrism. The evidence accumulated in the research network my work stands on regarding the God question is in my view as convincing as the evidence that supports heliocentrism and an Earth that is an oblate spheroid wobbling in precession. The evidence for a radically social brain, on the other hand, like the evidence for gravity and time, is somewhat more volatile.

The Body Information

The body is a boundary object between information and control in an era of bioinformatics. We have been witnessing a shift from a cryptographic to a pragmatic paradigm in biological discourse, and the emergence of hybrid bodies. The general process has been a commodification of the body, something we should recognize in more general terms as part of the commodifying blitzkrieg of latter-day "capitalism" (the economy that never was and never could be; Restivo, 2018: 186–93). Consider, for example, Robert Mitchell's (2004) views on body wastes, information, and commodification. We are living in transitional economies organized around informational modes of production. As we informaticize objects, bodies, and relationships, everything becomes more readily commodified, including body parts and body wastes. The global economy, as discourse and information, reaches its apex (as a system of inclusion and exclusion) in commodity imperialism, colonialism, and market expansionism.

New forms of embodiment abound; for example, in the form of virtual informatic surgeons, digibodies (a third space between mind and body), and informatic emotions. Finally, we find ourselves at the intersection of bioinformatics and the visual arts, engaging installations such as "Einstein's Brain" (Dunning, Woodrow, and their collaborators) and Kac's "Genesis." Here are the results of moving from conceptual criticisms of biotechnology to using it in aesthetic formations. A cult of information arises out of a sea of media bodies, reality-transforming symbols, and the mindbody (Hansen, 2015: 162) concept. The meaning of the human genome is not simply the province of scientists but a boundary object batted about and battered in the arenas of art, science, and culture. As we move through this world, representation fades away and data is made flesh. Simultaneously, the flesh becomes more complicated.

Nietzsche (and certainly our own contemporary students of body) helped make a place for new kinds of bodies, with new kinds of lives. It is in our (will to) power to construct new bodies, new entities, and new forms of life and kinds of lives. Bodies are systems of meaning, of interpretations, and this means that what counts as a "body" is a cultural decision. One could easily imagine that we are witnessing the end of the body. Claude Levi-Strauss (1967) argued that academics tend to focus their attention on things just at the point they are coming to an end. On closer inspection, however, endings are more likely to be transitions and transformations. This is implied, for example, in Martin's (1992: 121) contention that one sort of body is coming to an end and another kind of body is coming into being. In an era of postmodernisms, it is more prudent to think in terms of plurals rather than singles. Just as we are cautioned in science studies to think in terms of sciences instead of science (or Science), so we should be prepared to think of the body, and especially the emerging body, as bodies. This is simply the best of postmodernism at work, pluralizing our classifications and categories. The body, always in fact the focus of a pluralizing discipline if we think about it in historical cross-cultural terms, is arguably at the center of more intense disciplining actions than ever before. One reason is that the body is centrally linked to all the other entities now being subjected to pluralizing disciplining. This has implications for how we think about brains, which is why we need to consider these issues.

Judith Butler (1993) expressed her frustration with how resistant the body is to being disciplined. In order to get some purchase over her subject (and perhaps over her own body, her own self), she adopted a Foucauldian posture to address the regulatory norms through which the body is materialized. She found herself engaging with constructivism and questions about agency, but she problematized these ideas contra constructivism (or "constructionism," as I prefer) in a way that was prohibitively narrow sociologically. Notice that pluralization and disciplining impose new restraints and regulations on bodies and simultaneously provoke multiple forms of bodies (e.g., transgendered and trans-sexed bodies, and LGBTQ+, homo-, hetero-, and trans-normative relationships).

In *How We Became Posthuman*, Katherine Hayles (1999) analytically distinguishes the body from embodiment. Like many of us who are struggling to escape dualistic thinking, Hayles found it difficult to stay the pluralist or holistic course. More recently, she tried to complete her escape by adopting the strategy of positing "relation" rather than preexisting entities (on relational thinking as a recurring intellectual strategy, see Restivo, 1983: 40–41). She adopted Mark Hansen's term "mindbody" to denote the emergent unity of body and embodiment in a dynamic flux of biology, culture, and technoscience. The relational stance gives us mind, body, and world as constructions of our experience (Hayles, 2004; *cf.* Clark, 1998; Noë, 2010; and Restivo, 2017: 33–34).

The body as subject and object is a locus of tensions that emerge around new technologies. The powers behind these technologies announce them as gateways to utopias—it was atomic power in the mid-twentieth century. Later in that century, it was the human genome. And then bio- and nanotechnology. Since the 1990s, it has been the neurosciences. These announcements call forth critics who respond with dystopic and doomsday scenarios. As the *body technology*, increasingly fluid and evasive, emerged in the last century, Wells, Kafka, Orwell, and others imagined the dark futures that might lie ahead of us (Dyens, 2001). Today, authors such as Don DeLillo, Caleb Carr, Dan Brown, and Michael Crichton oppose the utopias of the utopitechnologists and the utopinformation engineers with visions of bodies and cultures transformed darkly in near-future dystopias.

When Oswald Spengler wrote in the 1920s that there is no Mathematic, only mathematics, he foreshadowed the emergence of ethnomathematics and helped usher in a world of multicultural pluralities and multiplicities. In this (brave?) new world of pluralities, even the bodies and identities of children are at stake. What sorts of children will come from a world in which the forms of family life, sexual and gender identities, and relationships are multiplying side by side with novel child-machine images? The future holds new ways of inscribing the body with desires and erotics, and the uncertainty of what lies ahead means the end of (depending on how much reality you ascribe to the Freudian notion) the Oedipal child (Poster, 2004) and the Jungian Electra child. What will happen to Jocastas? Perhaps we are harvesting the lessons about children and humanity we have been taught by history (e.g., in the work of Phillipe Aries) and imagined in science fiction (notably in Arthur C. Clarke's *Childhood's End*).

Pluralities and multiplicities do not mean that the future will be messier than the past. Unities, dichotomies, and trichotomies are connected to dimensional shifts. Things become multidimensional and blossom into pluralities and multiplicities; pluralities and multiplicities in many dimensions eventually resolve into unities that provoke polarities, the multiplication of dimensions, pluralities and multiplicities again, and so on. Life in this sense is cycles and spirals of thesis, anti-thesis, synthesis, thesis, anti-thesis and on and on. What drives this process is the innate dialectical nature of living things, and indeed things in general.

The late twentieth century may have ushered in the Age of the Body, the era in which echoes of Plato's complaints about the body finally faded away and thinking men and women began to rally around Nietzsche's claim that there is only body. All efforts in the post-Phaedo world to dissociate minds and brains from bodies have failed. Today, what remains of the Platonic vision and its transcendental progeny have become victims of the embodiment movement. What is this but the triumph of materialism(s)? We need to mobilize efforts that reject transcendence and eradicate vulgar versions of materialism without rejecting materialism.

Marx brought the calculus down to earth; Spengler and Wittgenstein went further and anthropologized mathematics. Durkheim is the modern locus classicus for the general rejection of transcendence. He is known for the argument that God is a collective formation and a collective elaboration—a symbol of society. What is not so well known is that, in the closing pages of the study in which he argues that God is a social construction, Durkheim also demonstrates that logical concepts are social constructions. With the coming of science studies and cultural studies we disciplined mathematical and scientific knowledge as cultural and social constructions. The next phase of this rejection of transcendence is now underway in the sociology and anthropology of mind and brain (e.g., Restivo, 2019). The final phase comes with the sociology of the gods, religion, the supernatural, and transcendence itself (Restivo, 2021).

Information has classically been as recalcitrant as mathematics and logic in resisting embodiment and materialization, but now it, too, is falling under the disciplining regimes of embodiment and materialism. The Age of Information might be enveloping the Age of the Body, even as both fall under the umbrella of the Age of the Social (Restivo, 2018).

R. Doyle (2004) affords us another opportunity to consider what is at stake in the informatic understanding of life by linking LSD and DNA narratives. He asks: What if Timothy Leary and Francis Crick were speaking the same language? The language of information becomes a locus of the organic and the machinic (or mechanic) enfolding each other helically, with the result that sometimes "the capacity for replication goes through the ceiling." Imagine this as at one with the cycles and spirals of thesis, anti-thesis, and synthesis and you have some idea of the roots of the complexities of life forms and technological forms. Doyle perceptively infers a Nietzschean joyous science (or science of joy) from life as information. He comes very close to embracing my claim that the best science is practiced anarchistically and within anarchistic social formations. If life emerges at the edge of chaos, moreover, we may as well say that it emerges at the edge of information, life *is* informatic, and bodies are at once and already bodies of information. It is a relatively short step to recognizing where the "feeling" for the cyborg (Woodward,

2004: 194) comes from; embodiment is necessary for learning emotions and generating consciousness.

The possibility of "peaceful collaboration" between humans and other forms of artificial entities (collaboration between organic and inorganic machines) is dependent on the cross-species communication of the "caring emotions" (especially empathy and sympathy). We are at the threshold not simply of understanding the conditions for relating to machines but to other humans, and most generally to the Other. Success depends on everyone coming to the dance.

CONCLUSION

All of the visionaries imagining the Age of the Body and the Age of Information are haunted by the specter of the Age of the Social. They must turn around and face this terror squarely (as must we all) in order to ground embodiment and bodies in social discourses and social practices. We and everything we invent and discover are socially constituted; there is no other way for us to make our worlds than through our interactions with each other as socially constructed selves, as members of a species that is always, already, and everywhere social. Here is where we will find the resolution of the mind/body and mind/brain problems and the hard problem of consciousness. The turn to the body is a significant reply to the mistaken focus on neurons and genes as the seats of our humanity, our creativity, our consciousness. It is not brains and genes that learn and act, but an integrated informatic system that erases the conventional boundaries between brain, body, and world. We socialize this informatic system, not selves, persons, or individuals in the classical senses of these terms. We "inform" this system. Some move in this general direction is necessary if we are going to overcome the cults of the brain, the gene, and the body. This is the sort of thinking that crystallized into my model of the social brain (chapter 11).

All of this may be an exercise in futility. I am writing with the shadow of the Doomsday Glacier looming over the world along with a variety of other existential threats to life and to the planet itself. But we Nietzscheans are obliged to think and think and think and to write and write and write and to speak and speak and speak until our very last breaths, "to rage against the dying of the light," as Dylan Thomas sings, even if it were after all for naught.

Chapter 6

Genius Incorporated

THE GENIUS BRAIN

My study of the fate of Einstein's brain (Restivo, 2020) and the socially networked roots of his genius echoes Hélène Mialet's (2012) study of Stephen Hawking. Mialet identifies the human, material, and machine-based networks that are Stephen Hawking. Hawking, like Einstein, was widely portrayed as a bodiless, singular individual, nay, singular mind. Viewed through the lens of anthropology and sociology Hawking is seen as incorporated, materialized, and instantiating a complex network of machines and humans.

Albert Einstein has been described as using the power of his "own thoughts" in 1916 to predict gravity waves. A century later, gravity waves were detected using highly sophisticated technologies. These technologies were opposed to Einstein's "own thoughts," thus reinforcing the concept of Einstein as the "genius of all geniuses." When we go looking for Einstein the man, we find only a sacred scientific hero. When we inquire about his brain, which was removed during his autopsy in 1955, we find only a sacred scientific relic. Indeed, it would find a central place in a reliquary of science museum along with Babbage's brain, Galileo's fingers and thumb, Bentham's body, Pasteur's tomb, Italian anatomist Antonio Scarpa's head, and Newton's death mask and hair, all of which have been preserved and are on display at various sites around the world (Beretta et al., 2016). It's time to try to find Einstein the human being and see if there's anything he can teach us about ourselves and our brains.

The term "genius" rests on the concept of the individual as an entity that stands apart from society, history, and culture and is even outside of time and space. An element of the divine spins the genius right out of the world into a sacred space. It sets Einstein and his brain apart from the rest of us.

65

I introduced the concept of genius clusters in chapter 5. The clustering of creative periods that are crucibles for the formation of geniuses was already recognized by the Roman historian Paterculus (d. 31 CE). Periods of creative clusters appear predictably during times of rapid decline or rapid growth within civilizations. The findings on genius clusters converge with studies demonstrating that inventions and discoveries are in principle multiples, not singletons (Merton, 1961). New ideas, theories, and technologies emerge simultaneously in different places in more and less circumscribed regions and share a family resemblance. The particular version that prevails and the individual or team that gets credit for the discovery or invention hinges on negotiation, politics, public relations, personalities, connections, and in some cases (for example, the electrical engineer Nikola Tesla) the outcomes of patent disputes.

The very idea of genius is based on the myth of individualism and the concept of the "I," a grammatical illusion. In terms of its original meaning, genius brings ideas of deities and guardian angels into the internal engine driving extraordinary creativity. There is no such thing as the lone wolf genius. Every genius is a social network. The genius stands on the shoulders of a social network. That this has to be the case is grounded in four fundamental ideas: (1) genius clusters; (2) clusters are not random; (3) innovations appear as multiples; (4) humans appear on the evolutionary stage as always, already, and everywhere social. We are not born individuals who become social; we are social animals who become socially organized social beings.

Where in the notion of Einstein's "own thoughts" is there room for collaborations with Michele Besso and Michael Grossman during the construction of the general theory of relativity? Grossman helped Einstein with the geometry and the concept of tensors he needed to formulate the general theory. Where in the portrait of the lone wolf patent clerk who published the revolutionary 1905 papers is there room for others in a network of influences, from Newton to his first wife, Mileva Marić, and numerous former teachers, friends, and colleagues in the physics community? How does Walther Mayer, Einstein's assistant during his Unified Field Theory period, relate to Einstein's "own thoughts"? Where is the lone wolf in the Olympia Society, founded by Einstein in 1902 and constituted of Einstein, Maurice Solovine, and Conrad Habricht, private students he tutored? The group was in existence until 1905. Conrad's brother Paul and Lucien Chavan occasionally took part. And Mileva Marić often listened in but did not actively participate. Among other discursive activities they read and debated the works of Mach, Karl Pearson's *Grammar of Science*, Poincaré's *Science and Hypothesis*, J. S. Mill's *Logic*, Hume's *Treatise of Human Nature*, Spinoza's *Ethics*, other works of science and philosophy, and even such literary works as *Don Quixote*. Einstein, the self-styled *Einsplanner* (one-horse cab) was created by "Einstein priests" and in part by our cultural mythologies about genius. Highfield and Carter (1993: 6) see the revelations of letters published in the Einstein papers project at Boston University as revealing Einstein's "flaws." The title of their book is more to the point as a clue to Einstein as a social network: *The Private Lives of Albert Einstein* (and see Farrell, 2001, on "collaborative circles"). The surprise is not that Einstein worked with and depended on others; it is that Einstein *is* those others—they make up his social self. Does the label "genius" help us understand Einstein or is it merely a stimulus for untutored awe and worship?

How Should We Understand Einstein's Uniqueness?

Developments in neuroscience, epigenetics, and social network theory since the 1990s do not challenge Einstein's uniqueness. If, however, we add these developments to those in the social sciences we are forced to rethink the nature of his uniqueness. His uniqueness is not a matter of genes, neurons, quantum phenomena, or the biological brain. Developments in social brain research and studies of the self in social science point us in a different direction. They tell us that his uniqueness is defined by the uniqueness of the set of social networks he encountered as his life unfolded. And if his brain holds any clues to his creativity, those clues would be functions of how his social environment impacted the architecture of his brain; his dead brain could not tell a story of innate genius.

Einstein and His Brain

Albert Einstein died on April 18, 1955. For students and faculty in my science and engineering high school this was an auspicious event. What I remember about that day is an emotional tone. The day stood out for me the way the day that Franklin Delano Roosevelt died sat in my mind, the way I remembered the day Babe Ruth died. On April 12, 1945, I was a child of five, but I understood that something big had happened: the president had died. I remember the day was cloudy and the world outside our windows was gray. I experienced a hard-to-define heaviness all day. I worked out that heaviness by marching around the living room dinner table to a recording of my favorite march. I can hear the music in my mind, but I don't know the name of the march. I was almost eight when Ruth died on August 16, 1948. That night, some friends of mine and I went out to see if we could see his shooting star taking him to heaven.

On April 18, 1955, Dr. Thomas Harvey performed the autopsy on Einstein's body at Princeton Hospital in Princeton, New Jersey. Harvey decided on his own initiative to remove Einstein's brain. Einstein had left specific instructions that he be cremated. He didn't want his body or body parts to become relics of awe and worship. Harvey may have been influenced by the fact that Oscar Vogt and his wife Cécile, under orders from the Soviet government in 1924, had removed Lenin's brain in order to study the origins of political genius. So Harvey removed the brain, sectioned it, sliced it into microscopic slivers, stained the slices, and mounted them on slides. Nothing was known about any of this until 1978. Eventually, Harvey's slides became the object of widespread study in the neuroscience community. I will come to that story shortly.

One can already notice contradictions between those who claim that Einstein was destined to be a thinker and those who point out the influence of Einstein's father and uncles on the direction of his early intellectual life. It has been easy to make mistakes in reference when it comes to our selves and our brains; they seem to be introspectively transparent. Certainly, experience is in the end the final arbiter of what is going on in and around us. However, it is not individual experience that we rely on in science but the collective, intersubjectively tested experiences of a community of scientists over time.

Genius is a symbolic device. The concept's significance is cultural, not scientific. As a cultural concept it is colored by the dominance of men in our and most societies. The male color of genius is readily explained by the fact that the thread that holds the tapestries of science, brain, and self together is patriarchy. In the modern political economy of genius, meeting Einstein or Edison is like meeting a god. If Einstein's brain has a story to tell, it's not going to be a story about individual genius, but a story that unravels the myths of self and brain that bind and blind all of us.

Many experts who studied Thomas Harvey's slides found nothing unusual about Einstein's brain. One of the reasons seems to have something to do with the particular way in which Harvey stained the tissues. It didn't allow for reliably distinguishing varieties of glia cells (astrocytes, oligodendrocytes, and microglia). Studies of myelinogenesis in the era prior to the development of complex network theories were not on the neuroanatomists' radar. Myelinogenesis is the proliferation of myelin sheaths, the sleeves of fatty tissue that protect your nerve cells. Harvey and his experts gave short shrift to myelin. No investigator in more than half a century has taken on the daunting task of scrutinizing the microanatomy of Einstein's myelinated axons or dendrites. Counting the cells of Einstein's thalamus was considered too time consuming and not liable to offer any informative results.

Some differences between Einstein's brain and small samples of "normal" brains were found in some studies. These differences were contaminated by methodological and other flaws, and in the end could not be unequivocally associated with "genius." The studies of Einstein's brain proved in the end to be sterile. First, they were guided by the questionable assumption that the

mind was the product of the brain (neuroism). Second, they reflected dissocism, a term I introduced earlier. To review, it is the inability to "see" social
life as the locus of the social causes that shape our behaviors, emotions, and
thoughts. You can think of it as "social blindness" by analogy with the mindblindness characteristic of people with autism (Baron-Cohen, 1995). A third
bias affecting these studies was the fallacy of introspective transparency, the
idea that you have immediate and objective access to your own consciousness or mind. Finally, these studies were contaminated by a conspiracy of
mythologies: the myth of individualism, the myth of the brain in a vat, and
the myth of brain-centric thinking reinforced by gene-centric thinking. A
2006 study of Einstein's brain found a diseased brain rather than the brain
of a genius. Colombo (2006) and his colleagues criticized earlier studies of
Einstein's brain for their inconsistencies and doubted whether microscopic
neuroanatomy studies could ever prove useful.

Einstein's Genius Cluster

Einstein's 1905 papers come in the midst of a cultural flowering of ideas,
inventions, and discoveries across the full spectrum of the arts, humanities,
and sciences between 1840 and 1930. Einstein's "genius" cluster in physics
included such luminaries as Lorentz, Planck, Tesla, Emmy Noether, Marconi,
Poincaré, Westinghouse, Madame Curie, the Wright Brothers, and Edison.
The two great innovations in physics that would remain at the core of physics
throughout the twentieth and into the twenty-first century, relativity theory
and quantum mechanics, were born in the early years of the twentieth century.
Expanding the genius cluster to encompass music we can include such names
as Sibelius, Puccini, Debussy, Schoenberg, Stravinsky, and Charles Ives.
Innovations in literature include the rise of the novel, American transcen-
dentalism, realism, stream of consciousness, various forms of modernism,
naturalism, the growth of children's literature, and the Harlem Renaissance
of the 1920s. In philosophy, we have Wittgenstein's *Tractatus Logico-
Philosophicus* from 1918. The Vienna Circle of elite philosophers was active
between 1924 and 1936. And there was a sympathetic mutuality that linked
Cubism (represented by Picasso's *Les Demoiselles d'Avignon*, 1907) and
relativity theory. Both involved challenges to conventions regarding absolute
time and space. Stein associated her writing with Cubism and thus one might
say with a literary transform of the theory of relativity.

CONCLUSION

The period 1840–1930 witnessed a veritable Copernican revolution, the emergence and crystallization of the social sciences, broadly conceived to encompass sociology, anthropology, and social psychology. I've described this period as the first Age of the Social. The second Age of the Social occurred between 1930 and 1970. This period gave rise to the sociology and anthropology of knowledge, science, and belief. We are now in the third Age of the Social, an age characterized by studies of the deep inner workings of science and the construction of facts, truths, and objectivity. It is also an age that is witnessing the diffusion of social science perspectives across the disciplines, the media, and the public arena. This period will last until at least 2050, by which time sociology should be taking its place among the classic robust sciences physics, chemistry, biology, psychology, and economics.

At the end of the day, the most insightful discussion of Einstein's brain can be found not in the halls of science and philosophy but in TV land. On July 21, 1999, the David Letterman TV studio audience was allowed to ask "Einstein's brain" (a model brain in a beaker of green Jell-O) questions. They are told that due to Einstein's death in 1955, the questioner is addressing dead tissue. This comedic vignette does more for neuroscience than all of the papers and lectures on Einstein's brain. In the wake of this analysis, I was challenged by a friend to explain the genius of John Coltrane in terms of social networks. The result is the following chapter.

Chapter 7

Improvisation Incorporated

This chapter began as a conversation I had with a friend of mine who challenged the idea that we are our social networks. It illustrates some of the everyday challenges of thinking sociologically about individual creativity. In addition to rehashing our conversation, I am going to add some materials on the sociology of improvisation as a specific form of creative work that forms the foundation for applying my challenge: Give me a genius and I will give you a social network.

ALICE, AND ME, AND JOHN

My friend Alice is an applied anthropologist. She started things off by asking me if I thought jazz saxophonist John Coltrane's improvisations were "pure or contaminated by his social networks." The background for this question is that Alice had recently read my book, *Einstein's Brain*, in which I make the claim: Give me a genius and I will give you a social network. I replied that social networks don't contaminate us any more than our circulation system, liver, or skin contaminate us. They are part of who and what we are and, like our liver or heart, are subject to pathologies. This goes to Alice's next question: Do you think social networks are only positive? She asked me if I knew anyone who ever murdered someone, or did I know anyone who had spent years in prison. I assume that humans are defined by the history of the social networks their lives unfold through. We *are* our social networks; we are always, already, and everywhere social. So, asking if social networks are only positive is like asking if our skin is only positive or if our limbic system is only positive. It doesn't matter whether you are Mr. Rogers, Hitler, Albert Schweitzer, or Mata Hari. They are all their social networks and their behavior, thoughts, and emotions reflect the history of the social networks their lives unfolded through. It's networks all the way down. However, just as our organs or cells can let us down and become diseased, social networks can also exhibit social pathologies.

Having come this far you will recognize that Alice, who is not naïve about society and culture, is still uncomfortable with the idea that we *are* our social networks. Clearly, this was not introspectively transparent to Alice, who is a professional social scientist.

In her book *Hawking Incorporated* (2012), Hélène Mialet's argues that in the twenty-first century, the idea of the cyborg is more reality than classic science fiction. We are all, as I have pointed out, networked socially but also, as Mialet shows, networked technologically: connected, extended, wired, and dispersed. Where is the individual, the person, the human, the body, or where do they stop, where are our boundaries? We are forced to consider these questions in a dramatic manner when confronted with Stephen Hawking, a man who was permanently and publically visible as a human being attached to assemblages of machines, devices, and social networks.

Alice and I then traded remarks about our knowledge of jazz. I said I know a little bit about jazz improvisation. I have a son who is a professional jazz musician and a professor of jazz. And sociologists have written quite a bit about jazz. Sociologist and semi-professional jazz musician Howard Becker has made notable contributions to the sociology of jazz. These contributions are part of his research on the world of art as a collective enterprise (Becker, 1982; and see https://jazzstudiesonline.org/jazz-topic/anthropology-and-sociology). Alice pointed out that she lived with a musician for forty years, a violinist who also played kanoon in an Arabic orchestra. So we could both claim to know something about improvisation. I am, incidentally, an amateur musician (piano and chromatic accordion, guitar, and piano).

In keeping with my emphasis on the invisibility of social causality, I pointed out that improvisation as a social network phenomenon is not obvious. Being a musician doesn't give you transparent access to the sociology of music. We then childishly traded some name calling.

What I know, I said to Alice, doesn't come from being a jazz musician. I'm only a reporter. I raised a jazz musician/professor, who taught me that improvisation is networked and programmed. It turns out this is what the research shows. That's what I relied on in replying to her Coltrane question. I asked her if there is an alternative research community on this question I'm not aware of. Was this her subjective sense of things, independent of any research-based data?

I then asked her why she asked the Coltrane question in a way which seems to presume an answer. She replied:

The thing is, Sal—it's obvious that Coltrane and all musicians use what they learned about chords, melody, patterns . . . but his individual creativity enabled him to improvise . . . such as in "Giant Steps" where he changed chords faster than anyone had before. He also improvised arrangements like beginning with a drum solo and ending with fast and furious playing. So through his own passion, his personal tone distinguishes him from others. . . . They all know the chords, patterns, etc., but he offers his personal insight—feeling. . . . Listen to "A Love Supreme"—have you heard anything else so amazingly personal? In some of his playing he revs up his sax and remains at that pitch to the very end . . . he keeps changing the melody in different ways. The point I'm trying to make is that Coltrane follows his breath—like the shakuhachi player—and keeps it flowing until he decides to stop. . . . My question is how does his individuality 'take' him to something different from others. . . . Yes he arrived at his monster saxophonist way through everything he learned—and yet changed it in a way that changed jazz. How does that fit into your theory of we are our networks?

We *are* our social networks the way we *are* biological and thermodynamical systems. But we all flow through life encountering different things, ideas, environments, people, and cultures. Those differences, as parts of the social networks our lives unfold through, are the differences that add up to our unique behaviors, thoughts, and actions. The fact that Django Reinhardt lost the use of the third and fourth fingers of his left hand meant that his social network expressed itself through him differently than it would have if he hadn't lost the use of those fingers. Art Davis had his fingers caught in a car door. His broken finger forced him to invent new techniques (Ratliff, 2007: 191). Sometimes it's a matter of having trouble with an instrument. In alto sax recordings in 1946, Coltrane's rhythms are awkward; he plays "short phrases with swallowed notes and woozy slides." This may be a reflection of having problems with his saxophone, of not being able to get the instrument to "speak instantly" (Porter, 1999: 45): "For example, on 'Embraceable You,' there are two places where his middle E doesn't speak, causing disturbing gaps in those phrases."

This shows that accidents of birth or in life, in technology, in context change the material that social networks work on. And accidents are *one* way our life course and the nature of our creativity work themselves out. Being born blind doesn't change the fact that you are a biological entity, but it changes the biology social networks work on and therefore impacts your behavior differently than if you were sighted. Just as mutations can show up in our DNA, biological, physical, and chemical changes ("mutations" by analogy) can show up in our bodies. These then to different degrees change the material social networks work on. The mutations can be more or less impactful. Whatever we are as original organisms and whatever we become, we never escape the laws of physics, the laws of biology, the laws of chemistry, or the laws of social networks.

The more dense, larger, and more complex our social networks become and the more complex our cultures and environments become the more open we become as human systems. Open systems are by definition *not* deterministic, *but* they are lawful (see Bohm, 1957). My failure to clarify this from the very beginning probably contributed to what was hanging us up, but I'd pointed this out in every one of the things of mine she'd read.

Since the density, size, and complexity of social systems increase over time, individuals and social orders become less predictable but never unlawful in the scientific sense. And yet because we are systems of systems, some systems or subsystems are more closed than others. So in fact there are a lot of things you can predict about human likes and dislikes based on class, sex, gender, education, etc. At the same time, the degree of openness in our systems and subsystems is an obstacle to prediction.

Sociology and Jazz Improvisation

Classically, creativity, or creative genius, has been explained in terms of genetics or brain science ("innate" gifts) or providential interventions (the guardian angel concept associated with the origin of the concept of genius, or the concept of a muse). The creative artist seems to embody indecipherable natural or mystical laws and random intersections of lines of causality that resist being disentangled. For some observers/listeners, improvisation seems to involve unforeseeable outcomes which are at the same time experienced as inevitable. This suggests the kind of compelling outcomes associated with logic. There is an aura in improvisation that suggests "anything goes," that jazz musicians get up on stage and play whatever they want, any way they want. The pathway toward a more realistic understanding of the structural constraints and patterns that determine improvisation in practice begins by adopting an ethnographic approach to jazz.

It's important to see creativity as a labor process. We are fortunate to have for reference studies of jazz by sociologists who are themselves jazz musicians, notably H. S. Becker (2006). Becker addresses the concept of "the work itself" and concludes that there is no such thing. All we have are the many occasions in which a work is performed, read, or viewed. Becker is the author of "the Principle of the Fundamental Indeterminacy of the Art Work." The sociology of art is the study of how works are made and remade. The creative act is a labor process and a collective one at that. Nonetheless, the myth of individualism continues to drive efforts to explain improvisation in jazz, including the use of Bayesian methods (Menger, 2006: 48).

The idea that improv is spontaneous and indeterminate does not mean it isn't lawful, which is the case for an open system. The "ordinary activities" of "organized imagination" are just the beginning of getting to the collective work that grounds the improvisation. For those who think of jazz improv as an "anything goes" phenomenon, they should be curious to learn that it can be taught. Improvisers can and do formalize the fruits of their studies and experiences in method books, teaching tapes and videos. "Free jazz," Jason Bivins (2015: 180) argues, "is a misleading description for music deeply shaped by African culture. Improv cannot involve just playing whatever you want whenever you want." It's a matter of being controlled by your subconscious self, things you're not aware of. This is a pathway for the sociologist to the sets of social networks that configure the subconscious. Some jazz musicians and other artists recognize this at some level. When drummer Art Blakey says that something moves from the Creator (God) to the artist to the audience, he is describing himself as a vehicle for a musical thought collective. Contrabassist William Parker is more specific: the free improv musician is a vehicle for the Creator's vibration (Bivins, 2015: 187, 206, 211, 222). The "Creator" is the mistaken reference for society, for social networks.

It is a mistake to link "improvised" with "unprepared" (Torrance and Schumann, 2019: 256). The improvised performance is the outcome of extensive advanced planning, and much of such a performance is played from sheet music. Musicians may agree beforehand on how long a specific passage of improvisation should last. They might agree on a fixed number of repetitions of a chord progression, a fixed number of bars, or a specific signal to indicate when it is time to resume an already-composed section. There are of course free jazz performances in which all the preset parameters are dropped. Prep time in jazz improv significantly overlaps with performance time.

One aspect of the network insight comes up in Richard Cave's (2000) concept of the "motley crew" challenge. The challenge is to select, coordinate, and sequence the activities of a band. The selection criterion is that members must be reliably committed to their professional skills.

Another feature of network consciousness is Coltrane learning in great company as he developed through the late 1940s and early 1950s. He began to assert the creative forces of the networks of those years, especially in the context of and following his work with Miles Davis. Dolphy and Coltrane expressed their love for music by constantly discussing histories. Critic John Tynan called their music (and Coleman's) the "New Thing," a function of that group's self-conscious efforts to "escape conventional improvisational schemes" (Bivins, 2015: 173). Their ability to achieve this was a function of the novelty of the jazz and musical networks they'd traveled through.

The basic conclusion we need to grapple with is that jazz improv is "a very structured thing that comes down from a tradition and requires a lot of thought and study" (jazz great Wynton Marsalis, quoted in Berliner, 1994: 63). Jazz musicians have a "variety of teachable, learnable improv techniques:

accentuations, vibrato dynamics, rhythmic phrasing, tonguing subtle bends, and other microtonal melodic inflections" (Berliner, 1994: 66–69).

There are three basic theoretical frameworks we can turn to in order to explain a creative activity like improvisation at the individual or collective level: tinkering theory of evolution and scientific practice, blind variation and selective retention, and iteration. Iteration is suggested by Berliner's (1994: 146) observation that jazz musicians "treat a formerly mastered phrase as a discrete idea"; they incorporate melodic patterns and chord voicings from classical composers such as Bach and Beethoven (Berliner, 1994: 118; and see Ratliff, 2007: 242). Jazz pianist Walter Bishop Jr. describes the process as imitation to assimilation to innovation (Berliner, 1994: 120). Musicians will also "synthesize personal discoveries with the most useful ideas gleaned from other players" (Berliner, 1994: 169). Coltrane's "Giant Steps," for example, became an "active vocabulary platform for improvising" (Berliner, 1994: 130). From the perspective of the individual, creative potential is related to how much musical cultural capital he or she accumulates and how diverse the capital is. Culturally, the jazz community has generated innovations by incorporating a melting pot of musical styles including ragtime, brass bands, spirituals, blues, classical, gospel, and reinterpreted standards from Gershwin and others. Spiritual and religious influences have played a big role in the history of jazz as demonstrated by Bivins (2015) in his book *Spirits Rejoice! Jazz and American Religion.*

Influences in jazz have been drawn from Europe, Africa, Cuba, Brazil, the Middle East, Jamaica, and India. Sonic ideas have been drawn from the everyday world of animals (e.g., wolves and whales), trains, and cars. Individual musicians have added idiosyncratic influences from childhood: walking home from church with a cousin, listening to his or her habit of humming tunes; listening to friends' renditions of soul music; listening to household recordings, rhythms, and meter from popular dances; hand clapping patterns during church hymns; watching the Ballet Africane in New York City; and listening to rock sounds and rhythms and hip-hop. These include some of the influences on Miles Davis. John Coltrane fused Broadway music into a jazz waltz, "Sound of Music." Improvising a solo based on the chords of an earlier tune describes, for example, saxophonist Lester Young's improvisations on the chords of "Lady Be Good." Jazz musicians routinely evaluate each other's inventions and innovations and share ideas and opinions with their social networks (Ratliff, 2007: 243, 285, 289, 446, 484). They begin to encounter the challenges of arranging music with their earliest experiences in group settings. Performers strengthen their musicianship and deepen their knowledge of jazz conventions as they move from band to band. The atmosphere of venues and the character of audiences are also factors that shape improvisation in conjunction with the circumstances of every recording session.

Bivins (2015: 22, 44–49, 117–19, 153–54) argues that what is compelling about jazz is "its historically identifiable resistance through improvisation, through its religiosities, to closure as part of its pursuit of the sacred"; jazz rituals resonate with ritualized improv in American religion. Examples are easy to come by: guitarist David Fiuczynski on the improvisational stimulation of the "fluidity of Taoism," saxophonist Bobby Zankel on Buddhism and improv, and Dizzy Gillespie on the influence of Baha'i and his general belief that music comes from "the world beyond." Sonny Rollins is less directly spiritual and more so at the same time: he says his music is his yoga; playing the sax is doing religion. Coltrane, as part of his wide-ranging study, explored Yoruban musical idioms.

Students of jazz put the lie to the "anything goes" myth by stressing the remarkable and rigorous training that provides the foundation for improv. There was always order, always theory, always carefully thought-through processes. Coltrane stands out in this respect. Besides following the principle of practice, practice, practice and studying various musical traditions (including religious ones), he was a careful student of the *Thesaurus of Scales and Melodic Patterns*. The chord changes in "Giant Steps" were "the stiffest exercise he has as yet given himself as an athlete of improvising." The chord changes were twice as fast as those Ray Noble used in "Cherokee." The tempo of "Countdown" was faster still than that in "Giant Steps." "It was frightfully controlled music" (Berliner, 1994: 130).

Improvisation has been described by musicians in colorful metaphors: "Prehearing an idea, grabbing onto it, and following it like chasing a piece of paper being blown across the street" (Berliner, 1994: 49, 189–90,); Coltrane and Wayne Shorter "talked about improvising and language. . . . Start a sentence in the middle, then travel backward and forward, toward both the subject and the predicate simultaneously."

The Work Itself

A lot of what passes for the analysis of jazz work is based on descriptive analyses that have a lot in common with the practice of ethnomethodology. In brief, ethnomethodology is a form of sociological analysis that focuses on how individuals use everyday conversation and gestures to construct a common sense view of the world. By relying on jazz musicians themselves to "follow the musicians" in order to understand what is going on, theory is eschewed and the problem of improvisation tends to be approached through a sort of "natural accountability." Ethnomethodology, in other words, stays close to the realities of folk sociology. Jazz improvisation, like logical reasoning under the ethnomethodological lens, is its own explanation. It's impossible to learn anything about the history and development of improvisation using this method. The problems that follow are a mirror image of those associated with the ethnomethodology of mathematics (Bloor, 1987). All that "natural accountability" achieves is to inform us that improvisation is accomplished in the course of some musical work. The question is: How does the local work of the jazz musician produce a result that appears to reflect the idea that "anything goes?" In logic this leaves us with a mysteriously compelling "transcendental" result. In jazz it leaves us with Creator, religious, spiritual, and ineffable results. What we have already seen is that by applying a little theory (eschewed by ethnomethodology and the myths of individualism and ineffable genius) we can begin to throw some light on the local creation of improvisation and deny that it comes from worlds beyond our own.

We can't just do jazz to explain improvisation; we are obliged to reflect on the process, to theorize it. This is the direction I have been taking us in by drawing attention to cultural capital, iterations, social networks, and the sociological implications of seeing oneself as a "medium" or "vehicle."

There has been some research on applying an evolutionary two-stage mental process to creative ideation based on Campbell's (1960) model of blind variation and selective retention (BVSR). Once again, this theory is applied at the level of the individual creator, who is viewed as the agent for mutating an idea, exploring various expressions of the mutation, and selecting the fittest variant. This process is repeated until a useful creative idea is constructed. Perhaps the leading exponent of this theory is Dean Simonton (2012). Liane Gabora (2013) notes Simonton's claim that ideas are generated through trial and error in large numbers. Simonton points to false starts, backtracking, and similar actions to support his trial-and-error thesis. Of the variants generated by the trials and errors, some are selected and some are rejected.

Gabora points out that "selectionism" and the changes it leads to operate from generation to generation; it is not intragenerational. Blind variation and selective retention does not include an inheritance mechanism. Simonton loosens the claims of chance or "quasi-random" variation, which makes BVSR consistent with the data on creativity but incompatible with Darwinian theory. The generation of creative ideas is biased away from randomness by expertise, logic, and the activation of remote associations. It is such biases that are causing change. Creativity involves the conscious elaboration of blindly generated variations into finished products. But sharing these variations with others is transmitting acquired traits. This means selectionism is inapplicable. It is applicable in principle if accrued changes are erased at the end of each generation. Lifetime changes transmitted to offspring drown out the slower population-level Darwinian mechanism of change. In addition, "the generation of one idea affects the conception of the task, and thus the criteria by which the next is judged. Therefore, successively generated ideas cannot be treated as members of a generation, and selected amongst. Thus not only is the notion of blind variation problematic with respect to the creative process but so is the notion of selective retention" (Gabora, 2013: 14).

On the other hand the BVSR approach, Gabora writes, has offered us some insights in our efforts to understand the creative process. Some examples that might yield to this sort of analysis could come from the new era of jazz in the late 1930s that saw increased use of the sixth and ninth degrees of the scale. 2–2–4 bar phrases were broken up, and motifs lasting three to four bars were experimented with at unusual places in song structures. It is not at all unusual to hear improv described in terms that evoke BVSR: "exploratory search of concerted variation on a firm foundation of known routines, shared rituals, and proven practices" (Faulkner, 2006: 96).

The Concept of Shedding Culture

Improvisation is work grounded in preplanning and precomposing ideas, designs, and shapes coupled with "unanticipated ideas conceived, shaped, and transformed under the special conditions of performance"(Faulkner, 2006: 92, 94–98). Shed culture exploits routines—it's about learning songs, scales, and arpeggios; playing musical lines over and over; and imitating and exploring restraints inside and outside of yourself, searching for your own sound. Then comes the process of shedding that culture: "The isolated work of shedding becomes responsive to cooperative behavior at work in a community of other musicians." (Becker et al., 2006)

Shedding is the study of the work behind the "work itself." Faulkner's principle of exploration and exploitation, his concept of shed culture and shedding, is yet another contradiction of the idea that "anything goes" in jazz. Faulkner, following Becker, reminds us that jazz musicians work together ("night after night") on a core of basic elements—chords, harmony, rhythm, motifs constantly repeated in various places. They experiment endlessly with choices that eventually become "inventions" and "innovations." This sounds like the tinkering principle in evolution and science (see chapter 3).

In considering the application of various theories to jazz improvisation we must consider the variety of creativity endeavors. Some commissioned works come with such specific regimens that the artist does little more than execute commands. The creative process at the extreme in this case is well defined and routinized. Some works, by contrast, seek to be "'purely random' in the modes of automatic writing, algorithmic composition, 'dripping' with the work of editing—in which the arbitrary character depends, finally, on an initial determination to use only the least considered gestures and to correct or eliminate nothing." There is a third borderline case, completely fragmentary work "whose progress obeys no initial formula nor any progressively striving toward coherence." More work in this area must be done before we can determine whether and how BVSR might contribute to a theory of jazz improvisation (Menger, 2006).

The Hype of the "Age of the Brain" and Improvisation

The worldview of the "age of the brain" (Davis and Scherz, 2022) in an "emerging neuorsociety" (Restak, 2006) proclaimed by neuroscientists readily equates self and brain (Frank, 2009). This is supposed to shift the focus from individual psychology to a "chemistry and physics of the soul" (Stone, 1997: 360). This matters because understanding our strange, allegedly computational brains sheds light on who and what we really are and how this translates into social policies (Eagleman, 2015: 1). It bears on the hows whys and whats of fighting, loving, educating, truth and knowing, social policy, and designing our bodies for the future.

The domain of creativity, and in particular the act of improvisation in jazz, has not escaped this neuro-mythology. For example, Limb and López-González (2012) focus their studies on the neural bases of artistic innovation, including jazz improvisations. These sorts of studies have "demonstrated" that musical creativity is not localized in one brain area but rather involves deactivating and activating different brain areas. Rosen et al. (2020) present results that support the idea that creativity is explained by a dual-process model: experience influences the balance between executive and associative processes. The functional neuroanatomy of creativity depends on how creativity is defined: by quality of products or type of cognitive processes. Even studies that adopt more sophisticated models or theories, such as Torrance and Schumann (2019: 266), continue to be constrained by the myth of individualism. These authors focus in the first place on "the ways in which *temporality* is crucially bound up with improvisation in a mesh of different time scales, both as an artistic discipline and as a daily practice." Secondly, they attend "to the cognitive processes behind an improvising musician's expertise." Contrary to Dreyfus's (e.g., 2007) notion of absorbed mindless coping, the authors identify a "path of open-ended expansion [and sometimes transformation] of . . . mindful experiential relation with . . . doing. . . . Our account supplants Dreyfus's idea of the ego-less absorbed expert [as applied to improvisation] by that of a mindful (i.e., present in the moment) improviser enacting spontaneous expressions of herself." Theoretically, the authors route to a post-Dreyfusian analysis of improvisation embraces enactivist (Varela et al., 1991) and 4E (embodied, embedded, extended, and enactive) accounts of cognition and action. They argue for extending 4E to 5E by adding "extemporized." While in general they are oriented to an embodied theory of cognition and action, their approach is sociologically flawed in two ways: (1) they don't embody embodiment in social networks; and (2) their approach sustains a distinction between mind, cognition, and action (mind/body dualism) surpassed by Ryle's (1949) notion that the mind is just the body at work.

Networks of Jazz

When sociologist and semi-professional jazz musician Howard Becker describes jazz as "inherently social," he is trivially bringing jazz into the sphere of human activity unencumbered by the myth of individualism and the myth of innate genius as a trait that is in the genes or in the neurons. There have, in fact, been numerous efforts to apply social network theories and models to jazz. These generally stop short of the claims Randall Collins and I make about inventions and innovations arising in social networks, but they provide a foundation on which we could in principle carry out the requisite analysis. McAndrew et al. (2015: 217), following Becker and others, underscore the fact that jazz happens in jazz communities and jazz worlds that are essentially network structures. They thus offer a strong rationale for using social network analysis to explore and explain key features of jazz, including its culture of improvisation. Let's review some of the more interesting jazz network studies.

Heckathorn and Jeffri (2001, 2003) have carried out network studies of jazz musicians using a respondent-driven sampling method (RDS). This method has classically been used to study "hidden populations" (Heckathorn and Jeffri, 2003: 48). In such cases there is no list of population members, privacy issues are at stake, networks are informal, and the population is relatively small. They explored various forms of affiliations: principal instrument, musical style, professional activity, financial factors, race, demography, and network size. They found that the strength of connections in the network of jazz musicians was characterized by "considerable cohesion." It is important for readers new to sociology to recognize that social relationships are "conduits through which resources flow" (Heckathorn and Jeffri, 2003: 48). This is another way of saying what I mean when I describe the self as a configuration of the social networks one travels through in the course of one's life and work.

We have seen earlier the way the myths and cults of individualism and genius ground neuro-reductionist theories of improvisation. These studies tend to assume that musical improvisation is one of the most complex forms of creativity, an assumption I have no problem accepting. From one neuro-reductionist perspective, it is only possible because improvisers learn and reuse patterns of notes that they insert into the work of improvising (Vergara et al., 2021). Improvisation appears to involve a high degree of repeated musical patterns. Improvisers (again, keep in mind that the focus in this neuro-reductionist perspective is on the individual improviser) develop strategies for concatenating these reusable musical patterns that lead to new patterns of harmonics and rhythm. This may involve new playing (motor) movements and information about style and performance context.

This "improviser" is sociologically a social network, not an independent, free-standing individual whose brain is doing all the work. Of course, the brain is active during improvisation, and neuro-reductionism can indeed tell us something about what it is doing during improvisation. What Vergara et al. (2021) found was a specific brain network functionality involving two major networks: the default mode network (DMN) and the executive control network (ECN). This suggests a functionality that correlates idea generation (DMN) and retrieval and evaluation (ECN). Such studies will prove to be less reductionist when they can be incorporated into the sort of social brain network I argue for in this book.

Teitelbaum et al. (2008: 1, 12) analyzed community structures in two different social networks: similarity networks ("strong correlation between clusters of artists and musical genres") and collaboration networks (small-community structures related to bands and geographic zones, and larger communities based on "collaborative clusters with a large number of participants related through the period the artists were active"): "In the collaboration network . . . jazz players are the most active artists and give rise to the appearance of large communities related to different generations."

An examination of these collaboration networks shows that "high in-degree nodes" are famous jazz artists. In the era we're interested in the top-five jazz artists are Dizzy Gillespie, Duke Ellington, Miles Davis, Benny Goodman, and John Coltrane. High-pageview nodes are pop-culture celebrities (top-five: George Michael, Alicia Keys, Barbara Streisand, Liza Minelli, and Bing Crosby). This suggests the existence of a left–right polarization corresponding to a more or less pure-jazz lineage. The degree of a node in a network (sometimes referred to incorrectly as *the* connectivity) is the number of connections or *edges* the node has to other nodes. If a network is directed, meaning that edges point in one direction from one node to another node, then nodes have two different degrees: the in-degree, which is the number of incoming edges, and the out-degree, which is the number of outgoing edges (Venturini et al., 2021).

Kirschbaum and Ribeiro (2016: 1206–7) review the literature on the social aspects of innovation which stresses "spatial" metaphors. This literature has produced a major paradigm with twin ideas: "(1) core actors are more likely to introduce cumulative innovations, while (2) peripheral actors are more likely to bring disruptive innovations." This "core/periphery" dichotomy is challenged by research (Cattani and Ferriani, 2008) which shows "that boundary-spanners between core and periphery are more likely to introduce innovations into the field. . . . We have shown that the isolate actors in the

USA present higher odds of adopting a transgressive style when the field in which they are embedded is less centralized." This is not the case in Europe probably because of the greater centralization of musicians in European networks. Territories matter in the case of adopting new practices. Imposing a network layer on a territory helps us understand how actors in distinct roles will behave differently. Conversely, territories not only differ in degree of cohesiveness but also in terms of degree of hierarchical structures associated with different role structures. Joining the global jazz circuit makes it easier for the musician to throw off the constraints of conventional musicianship and adopt a transgressive style.

Vedres and Cserpes (2021: 1187) ask: What is the role of collaboration in innovation? The paradox of experience is that "successful teams need to build from the experience of members—and recording jazz requires considerable experience from musicians—while the team needs to avoid locking into routine solutions." They identify an equally paradoxical possible solution: network tension. This structural feature mobilizes the pursuit of new ideas in a team by way of an unbalanced network. Such a network is expected to push members apart. Under the influence of Aral and Van Alstyne (2011) and classically Granovetter (1973), the sociology of networks has been ruled by the principle of balance: strong ties are closed, open ties are weak. Vedres and Cserpes reconceptualize networks in terms of collective exploration and the local generation of new knowledge. Frequency- and strength-based measures of network tension consistently predict the creative success of teams. Open and weak triads, brokerage, or closure are mostly negative predictors of success. The authors review their findings in relation to several different potential explanations. These studies control for instrument diversity and level of experience. The inclusion of a brokerage variable would identify the presence of a central figure orchestrating network configurations. These controls allow the authors to empirically account for a large share of the variance offered by others attempting to account for the innovative success of a musical team's network. It is possible using the authors' simulation approach to estimate individual impacts on organization. Conscious effort reinforces lucky accidents. Unexpected tension is more likely to lead to successful creative efforts. The synergy of synchronous sound must cohere for new sounds to emerge.

Keith Sawyer (2008: x) writes about jazz what Randall Collins and I assume for all groups and networks: "in jazz the group has the ideas, not the individual musicians." Faulkner and Becker (2009: 185, 200) explain that players who haven't rehearsed sound like they have because they are brought together repeatedly in similar situations requiring the same kind of music: "They may not have rehearsed, but they have played the same things together many times, in various combinations, and thus have developed what might be called network-specific repertoires."

The non-obvious sociology of jazz "genius" is that individual musicians develop distinct styles by way of their lives unfolding through particular sets of social networks. Style, in other words, is not just a property of the individual. Network analyses tend to stop short of my sociologically grounded claim that networks are the locus of ideas, and individuals are vehicles for expressing those ideas, but they come very close (McAndrew et al., 2015: 227): "a band ensemble partly defines the musicians who belong to it, while each musician is individually defined by their network of band memberships." While their research is exploratory and methodologically limited, sociological theory offers a strong foundation for supporting the "strong but defensible assumption that the direction of causality does run from connectedness to success rather than the opposite."

Let's now return to Alice's question: She started things off by asking me if I thought Coltrane's improvisations were "pure or contaminated by his social networks." I explained that we *are* our social networks; we are not "contaminated" by them. To think that could lead us to argue that we are contaminated by our genes, our neurons, our skin, or our breathing apparatus. In reviewing key pieces of the literature on the social networks of jazz, I have established a rationale for my claim that John Coltrane *was* his social networks. The other piece of the sociology of genius theory is that we should consider whether there is a "genius cluster" associated with Coltrane. And indeed there is.

Coltrane's musical network begins with his family. His mother was a church pianist, and his father played the violin. He was also exposed in his early years to the music of the southern African American church. This influence manifested itself after 1960 when he took a "religious turn." This was also a period marked by the turmoil of the 1960s, and this era of cultural growth was necessarily characterized by confusing and confused paths across America and the world as people struggled to right the wrongs of civil society. Coltrane's music reflected this turmoil.

Network diagrams in Venturini, Jacomy, and Jensen (2021) show dense networks of jazz musicians constructed around the key nodes of Gillespie, Ellington, Coltrane, Davis, and others. They also construct networks showing linkages between jazz-rich periods in the 1920s, '30s and '40s, '50s and '60s, '70s and '80s and rock, country, progressive rock, RYB/rock, gospel and religious music, blues, hard rock, and standards. This is exactly the kind of dense multi-musical network we would expect in an era that was producing innovative jazz artists.

Just as in the case of Einstein, innovative professional and cultural networks abound in the growth-culture era from the 1920s to the 1960s and especially during the 1960s. We find important developments already emerging in the late 1950s. The Jazz Loft Project archived four thousand hours of recordings by major jazz artists playing in a Manhattan loft shared by D. X. Young,

Dick Cary, and Hall Overton. On December 8, 1957, *The Sound of Jazz* was broadcast live, setting a high standard for jazz television. The "A Great Day in Harlem" photo was published in *Esquire* magazine on August 12, 1958, showing fifty-seven jazz greats. Several key recordings in the history of jazz improvisation appeared in 1959: Miles Davis's "Kind of Blue," John Coltrane's "Giant Steps," and Ornette Coleman's "Shape of Jazz to Come." And Ellington recorded the soundtrack for the film *Anatomy of a Murder*.

The cultural-growth period from 1930 to the 1960s included "stream-lining," evolving out of Art Deco, and organic design (including Frank Lloyd Wright's organic architecture). There were ties to and echoes of the turn-of-the-century cultural-growth period (1900–1930) that gave rise to advances in science, technology, literature, and the arts period Einstein, Planck, Picasso, and Gertrude Stein thrived in and the cultural-decline period of the First World War. Surrealism (which would create links between Einstein and Magritte), abstract expressionism (Pollock), and later Pop Art (Lichtenstein, Warhol) and the foundations for postmodernism formed part of the context within which the inventions and innovations of jazz evolved.

CONCLUSION

The Jazz Machine

Perhaps the major insight we've uncovered in exploring improvisation is that it is not an "anything goes" phenomenon. It is structured. The extreme conclusion this insight gives rise to is that improvisation can be programmed. Before our review this would have seemed to lead to the oxymoron "programmed improvisation." And indeed, AI researchers have been exploring the possibility of AI jazz improvisation. Their starting point is the concept of the "social machine," a concept that has the scent of sociology. The contemporary meaning of *social machine* is an environment composed of humans and technology interacting and producing products and actions. At first glance, this sounds like Bruno Latour's actor-network theory (ANT). But it is not as well theorized. I discuss the nature and sociological limits of ANT in Restivo (2022: 161–88). The concept of social machine is also used in Randall Collins's (1992: 41) paradigmatic discussion of ritual and group behavior. He describes group meetings as energy transforming social machines: "By plugging into the group situation, individuals can make themselves stronger and more purposeful. This is the hidden payoff that accounts for the continuous appeal of religion and its secular equivalents."

The idea of AI improvisers is not as problematic as might at first appear. After all, we already have AIs that improvise jazz: human jazz musicians.

This is a counter-intuitive idea that requires understanding humans as organic machines. This is generally understood to mean that we are merely fleshy robots, biological machines. The trick is to see that we are organic, open systems, social machines—a perspective that follows from the opening chapters of this book.

In the case of the Carr and Zukowski (2018) experiment, a neural network was trained on Coltrane's "Interstellar Space" recording of 1967, modified with SampleRNN, an unconditional end-to-end neural audio generation model. The AI listened to the recording over and over for sixteen trials and then created its own musical piece.

It's easy to criticize such early innovations (e.g., *Virtual Reality Brisbane News*, 2021) but worthwhile, recalling the controversy caused by jazz fusion in the 1960s and '70s, which combined rock music and technology. From this perspective, AI-generated jazz looks like a "next step" and not a revolutionary move.

The social machine approach to AI jazz (Irvine and Cardo, 2019–2021) is based on the concept of jazz as "operations" (interactive improvisation) on "data" (song structures, rhythmic conventions, etc.). The social machine of jazz "aggregates the 'energy' of networked participants [data] and converts this via interaction into meaning." This approach is based on a sociologically viable concept of jazz improvisation as a function of complex social interactions. Improvisation is characterized in terms of annotating an original tune and situating the improv in that tune's history. The prospect of constructing an AI jazz improviser is daunting, even if it "knew" the complete history of jazz. The point to consider here is what the possibility of computerizing improvisation means for our common sense understanding of the creative genius of the improviser. My goal in this chapter has been to offer a rationale for the conjecture that improvisation has structure, pattern, and order and emerges in social networks, not individual brains.

Chapter 8

From the Matrix to Reality

ARE WE BRAINS IN VATS, SIMULATIONS, OR BRAINS IN THE WORLD?

The Matrix (1999) is a film about a future in which humanity is trapped within a simulated reality. The film draws our attention to two major ways in which philosophers have dealt with skepticism about our perception of reality: simulations, and brains in vats.

ARE WE BRAINS IN VATS?

The idea that we are brains in vats is a philosophical gloss on the idea that we are our brains. Cracks have developed in this paradigm, but it still dominates how philosophers, neuroscientists, scientists in general, and the lay public think about the brain. The idea has been written into the two main presidential proclamations on neuroscience in the last thirty years: President Bush's Decade of the Brain proclamation in 1990, and President Obama's BRAIN initiative in 2013. Both proclamations are based on the idea that the brain is the causal source of all of our behaviors, emotions, and thoughts.

The brain-in-a-vat (BIV) scenario is a common theme in science fiction. Louis Ulbach's "Le Prince Bonifacio" (1860, in *L'Isle des Rêves*) is one of the earliest examples of this genre. Well-known examples of BIV science fiction include stories by H. P. Lovecraft and E. E., Smith that appeared, respectively, in the magazines *Weird Tales* (1931) and *Astounding* (1950). The magazines *Wonder Stories, Fantastic Story Quarterly, and Galaxy* also published BIV stories in the 1950s and 1960s. Recent exemplars include Scalzi (2005) and Sanderson (2015). BIVs also appear in films (e.g., *Charlie Chan in Honolulu*, 1938; *Donovan's Brain*, 1953) and television ("The Gamesters of

Triskelion," a *Star Trek* episode, 1968; "The Brain of Morbius," a *Doctor Who* feature, 1978).

The BIV (also known as brain-in-a-jar) hypothesis is a thought experiment that reflects philosophical thinking about skepticism and solipsism. It was classically proposed by Descartes in his thoughts on an "evil demon" who deceives us about reality. The BIV idea appears in a modern context in Harman (1973/2016). It leads to an enormous literature on this thought experiment. Because philosophers are not constrained by the everyday world the rest of us live in, their speculations are guided only by the rules of logic, language, and imagination. There are no stop signs in philosophical discourse. The philosophical game includes in part exploring the many ways we can put sentences together logically and linguistically. A good thought experiment in physics is a mental exercise that has some roots in real physics and that could in principle be tested in the real world itself or lead to a relevant laboratory experiment. Thought experiments in philosophy are not under the same constraint. I am skeptical of the uses of philosophy once we have the methods and metrics of science. Therefore, I view the BIV as a luxury only philosophers have access to, and only philosophers can make hay with. Since this is one of my basic foils in arguing for the social brain, and since it is overtly and covertly at work in neuroscience, science at large, the media, and the public arena, let's see what it's all about.

The BIV idea reflects legitimate impulses to think—indeed, to worry about—how we know and what we can be certain we know. The lines of thinking here all focus on the individual. Without the myth of the individual, this kind of thinking would sink into history's abyss of sterile ideas. The BIV thinker supposes that some entity removes your brain, suspends it in a life-sustaining liquid in a vat, and connects its neurons to a supercomputer. The computer sends signals to the brain in the vat that are identical to the signals it received in the outside world, thus simulating reality. The disembodied BIV is now having normal experiences of awareness and consciousness. One question should be whether, when the brain is removed, it becomes a tabula rasa which can be fed a simulated reality or it would retain original configurations from the real world that might interfere with or contaminate the new simulated signals. Before we consider the absurdity of this idea, let's consider some other illustrations of this logical game. We can trace BIV thinking to the Hindu Maya illusion, Plato's allegory of the cave, Zhuang Zhou's dream that he was a butterfly, and Descartes's evil demon.

Maya means magic or illusion in Sanskrit. It is a fundamental Hindu concept originally defining the power of gods to make humans believe in illusions. Philosophical extrapolation led to the idea that the world of our experience is in fact an illusion. There are further spiritual considerations that follow, but these just draw us deeper into the trap of philosophy without stop signs.

One of the most famous exercises in the history of epistemology is Plato's allegory of the cave. Epistemology is a branch of philosophy that asks what knowledge is, how knowledge is acquired, and how we know (and with what certainty) what we know. In science, it is simply the theory of knowledge and knowing. The allegory is reported in Plato's *Republic* (ca. 375 BCE). Socrates is explaining some ideas about knowledge and wisdom to Glaucon (Plato's brother). He asks Glaucon to imagine some people who are born and grow up in an utterly dark cave. They are chained and cannot move their bodies or heads. They can only see the wall in front of them. Socrates now constructs a scenario in which some other people light a fire behind the "prisoners" and project shadow figures onto the wall they are facing.

The prisoners now see shadow forms of objects, humans, and animals from the world outside the cave on the wall they are facing. Glaucon is asked to consider whether the prisoners would accept these shadows, the only things they know, as reality. He agrees. Now Socrates frees one of the prisoners, who turns around only to be blinded by the light and unable to see the objects whose shadows he has been seeing. The shadows appear more real to him than the actual objects and beings themselves. The light of the fire would also be so painful that he'd turn back to the darkness he has always known.

In the next scenario, Socrates takes the prisoner out of the cave into normal daylight, leading to greater confusion than when he faced the light of the fire. To avoid these experiences with the firelight and daylight, Socrates suggests accustoming the prisoner to the outside world, exposing him by degrees to the shadows, reflections of objects and living things in water, and finally to the objects and entities themselves. Once he adjusted to sunlight, he could begin to understand reality. Now Socrates returns the prisoner to the cave, where he tries to describe what he has seen and learned to the other prisoners. They would think he was blind and dangerous. They might even kill him if he tried to free them. Socrates now explains the allegory.

The darkness of the cave represents visual signals, the fire is the sun, and the outside world represents the journey of the soul from the regions of the shadows to the realm of intelligible reality. Once within the "world of knowledge" the former prisoner is able to explain ideas like "the good" and "justice" to those who had only seen shadows of the good and justice. We can skip over the further lessons Socrates offers Glaucon concerning the good ruler and the objective of education and enlightenment, never mind the nature of the shadow that would be cast by justice.

The *Zhuangzi* is a Chinese text from the Warring States period (476–221 BCE). The text, named for Master Zhuang, one of its authors, narrates the carefree life of the Taoist sage. It is one of the two foundational texts of

Taoism, the other being the *Tao Te Ching*. The most famous story in the collection is "Zhuang Zhou Dreams of Being a Butterfly." Upon waking after dreaming he was a butterfly; Zhuang Zhou was no longer sure if he was Zhuang Zhou the dreamer or a butterfly who had dreamed he was Zhuang Zhou. This is an aspect of the human condition we have all experienced when we have found ourselves uncertain about whether something we remember was a dream or something we experienced in our waking lives. How do we know whether we are dreaming or we are awake? Once again, as in the BIV and cave allegory, we have philosophers trading on the complexities of our waking and sleeping lives to sustain their employment. Unfortunately, this has tended to lead us down the rabbit hole of infinite discourse rather than into enlightenment and wisdom.

Descartes's demon appears in his 1641 *Meditations on First Philosophy*. He imagines an evil, malicious demon with great power and cunning committed to deceiving him. Descartes, at the mercy of the demon, experiences the external world as delusions of a dream world, a world in which he falsely believes he is a flesh-and-blood being. This is an extreme example of the method of systematic doubt employed in the *Meditations*.

The factual basis of these philosophical exercises is the human experience of dream worlds juxtaposed with real worlds, worlds of truth nestled in with worlds of falsehoods and subatomic and cosmic realities lying outside of everyday realities. Our world, our universe, is complicated. It is characterized by levels of reality, microcosms and macrocosms, and meta-philosophies such as the six realms of Buddhism. So, it was inevitable that thinkers would realize that getting to know things, figuring out how things worked, and ultimately distinguishing truths from falsehoods was not simple and straightforward. And so, the introspections and analyses began. This led to concepts like solipsism, simulations, and BIVs. The most reasonable outcome of these introspections and analyses was skepticism. There are two basic forms of skepticism: realistic or scientific skepticism makes us cautious about our scientific claims but doesn't close down scientific inquiries; irrational skepticism is so extreme that it can stop science in its tracks.

Solipsism is the idea that the only thing we can know for certain is our own mind. Extreme solipsism tells us we are the only thing that is real; everything and everyone else is delusion. We cannot be equally certain that anything at all exists outside of our mind. Full stop. Why would it ever occur to anyone to doubt the external world? For one thing, the external world is a constant and recalcitrant, irritating reminder that we are flesh and blood, and mortal. It has provoked philosophers and theologians from at least Plato on to wish for a fleshless mind or an eternal, immaterial soul. Pin this on the individual and you generate all sorts of spinoffs and ultimately the BIV. The BIV is a disembodied brain, a close cousin to the Platonic dream of a disembodied mind or soul. Solipsism can be dismissed as a failure of the sociological imagination that gives us the myth of individualism. Skepticism is a core ingredient of the scientific worldview. When restricted to the individual as a mythical entity it can give birth to BIV imaginings and questions about what it's like to think like a bat, a Martian, and even a vampire. Since there are no stop signs on the roads of philosophy, it is inevitable that philosophers will generate groundless thoughts and entertain themselves on these thoughts for decades if not millennia.

There are certainly reasons to question our experience and to inquire about—to stay with the philosopher's context—qualia. What is it like to have specific experiences as a human, a bat, or made-up entities like Martians and vampires? At this point philosophers have reached the edge of the cliff of reason and inevitably thoughts of bats, Martians, and vampires will push some of them over the edge. We can also in this context have conversations about indexicality (what time is it now and who am I?), and personal identity. So, is there anything to learn from the BIV thought experiment?

There are a number of substantive reasons to question the value of the BIV. The BIV is disembodied, therefore it cannot have the same experiences as a brain in a body in the world. The brain has connections to the body, the body has connections to the social world, and the social world is embedded in an environment populated by flora, fauna, and physical, chemical, and biological objects and processes. The counterargument is that a BIV could be made to replicate all of these connections. We already have such a machine—the human being.

The living brain has multiple interrelated sensors that receive and process a complex set of inputs from the world it lives in. Whatever is being input to the BIV could never replicate this system. The philosophy of BIV is an exercise in the fancy and fanciful manipulation of logic and language by people who are guided by the myth of individualism, the grammatical illusion of the "I," brain-centric thinking, and the fallacy of introspective transparency. This conspiracy of mythologies is a nice basis for interesting science fiction scenarios that can at best entertain us but cannot at the end of the day educate us about the nonfiction story of ourselves and our world.

Kant, under the influence of the conspiracy of mythologies, put into words the reigning strategy behind philosophy—that our knowledge of the world is synthetic, that it comes to us through language. It does not. Our knowledge comes to us through our socially and culturally mediated activities in the world. It is this fundamental flaw in philosophy that produces science fiction and makes it appear to be relevant to science or general intellectual inquiry.

Could We Be Brains in Vats?

There are three basic refutations of the brain-in-a-vat argument:

1. The BIV is just not like an embodied brain neuroanatomically or neurophysiologically and so could not have experiences "just like" those of an embodied brain. BIV advocates could counter that a machine could be built to replicate real-world inputs to a real-world brain. Where would it get the material for real-world inputs unless there were already a real world with real brains? This is a classic illustration of philosophy without stop signs.

2. An embodied brain exchanges inputs and outputs across a network that links the brain, the body, and the world the body acts in. The five senses are the pathways from world to body to brain. In the case of the BIV, by contrast, the supercomputer is connected to the neurons. This is known as the argument from externalism; BIV representation cannot reproduce embodied brain representation.

3. The best-known argument against the BIV comes from Hilary Putnam (1981: 1–21). The scenario, Putnam argues, is simply self-refuting. Skirting Putnam's use of "Twin Earth" and "a monkey types Hamlet" scenarios, Putnam's argument comes down to the fact that a BIV that exists only in a simulation could never say, "I am a brain in a vat." "Brain" and "vat" can only refer to things inside the simulation. If the speaker is not a BIV, the statement is also false; thus, the BIV scenario is self-refuting. But things don't end there because without stop signs there is always going to be a clever philosopher with a counterargument. In this case, for example, we can assume Putnam's reference theory but kidnap an embodied brain and place it in a simulation. The BIV could then refer to real brains and vats. But Putnam could counter that his argument applies to a "pure" BIV and not a kidnapped brain. Points and counterpoints go on and on and on. Critics counter Putnam, and Putnam supporters reconstruct Putnam's argument to fortify it. The critics return. And so on and so on. The only way to put an end to these endless scenarios and counter-scenarios is for sociologists and other scientists to put up stop signs.

Are We or Could We Be a Simulation?

The Matrix in the film of the same name was created by artificial intelligence (AI) machines in order to gain access to the energy of human bodies. The film *The Matrix* draws on several contemporary and classical images and philosophies to construct its dystopia. The philosopher Jean Baudrillard's book

Simulacra and Simulation (1981) appears on screen ("the book used to conceal disks") and the character Morpheus's remark "desert of the real" is taken from Baudrillard's book. Baudrillard has said that the film does not accurately portray his ideas. But accurate portrayal is not a goal in the creative arts.

Morpheus is devoted to finding the "One," the human destined to bring the Machine War to an end. Here we have the classical Frankenstein idiom of the machines we create turning against us. The political philosopher Langdon Winner (1977: 313) wrote about this in his book *Autonomous Technology*. The issue at stake in the Frankenstein story is "the plight of things that have been created but not in a context of sufficient care." This, of course, is true of humans: Milton (1674/2013: 200) said as much in *Paradise Lost* when he wrote: "Did I request thee, Maker, from my clay / To mould me man? Did I solicit thee / From darkness to promote me?"

The Matrix interweaves our classical concerns with out-of-control technologies with contemporary worries about AI singularities, projected moments when manufactured machine intelligence will exceed our own and pose existential threats to humanity. This is a recurring theme in science fiction, from *Frankenstein* (Mary Shelley, 1831/1994) to *Neuromancer* (Gibson, 1984) and the works of science fiction author Philip K. Dick (particularly Dick's *Exegesis* [2011]). In 1977, Dick told an audience at a science fiction conference in France, "We are living in a computer-programmed reality, and the only clue we have to it is when some variable is changed, and some alteration in our reality occurs" (Virk, 2019: 2). *The Matrix* is also adumbrated in Descartes's "evil demon," which poses the possibility that we are living in an illusory reality created to deceive us. And indeed, the film has been connected to the philosophy of the BIV.

The Simulation Scenario

The simulation scenario posits that we humans are living in a computer simulation. We are again in the realm of the Hindu Maya illusion, Plato's allegory of the cave, Zhuang Zhou's dream that he was a butterfly, and Descartes's evil demon. What could be behind this kind of thinking? What could prompt someone to actually assign a probability to the likelihood that humans are living in a simulation? Let's consider first how the simulation scenario differs from the BIV argument.

The BIV argument is essentially an argument designed to prompt us to be skeptical about what we know and how knowledge is possible. It is also conceivable that we could create something like a BIV in a laboratory. That is, we could conceivably keep a brain alive and get it to receive and send signals. The research in this area involves primarily "brain organoids." These are not real brains but rather three-dimensional structures grown from stem cells derived from actual adult human brain cells (Bardy et al., 2015; Gabriel et al., 2022; Gordon et al., 2021; Luo, et al., 2016; Reardon, 2020). But such a "brain" would not be a brain in a body in the world and therefore could not demonstrate any of our cognitive, behavioral, or emotional states. A simulation goes much further. It proposes that the world, the brain, life, the universe, and everything is a simulation. In the BIV scenario, the "person's" experience is exactly the same as the experience of the person in the world. In the simulation, reality and our subjective experience are reduced to illusions.

Philosophically, the most reasonable way to understand the BIV argument is as a metaphor. The simulation scenario is more explicitly a statement about the nature of reality. Some philosophers bolster their claims about simulation with probability estimates. Nick Bostrom, who introduced the simulation argument in a 2003 paper, argues "odds are" we are living in a simulation. Elon Musk has put the odds at 99.9 percent. This is numerology or metaphoric math, not mathematics. The historical grounds of Bostrom's argument rest, earlier contributions notwithstanding, in the classical contributions of Descartes's evil demon and the modern speculations by Hans Moravec (1999: 91) on simulation, consciousness, and existence. Moravec is an advocate of physical fundamentalism. Physical science is our only route to true knowledge. Other belief systems are just "made-up stories." And yet Moravec believes that physical fundamentalism is compatible with the Cartesian conjecture that the world of our perceptions is an "elaborate hoax."

What, then, is the source of these arguments? In Moravec's case they are a consequence of assuming physical fundamentalism. More generally, they arise and can be sustained only so long as we cannot solve the "hard problem" of consciousness. If we can solve the hard problem of consciousness, we eliminate the fuel that sustains BIV and simulation arguments. Such arguments are, however, also fueled by the "hard problem" of God. David Chalmers (Thomas, 2022) has explicitly identified a "programmer in the next universe up," implying a god or god-like entity: "[It] may just be a teenager," Chalmers said, "hacking on a computer and running five universes in the background. . . . But it might be someone who is nonetheless omniscient, all-knowing and all-powerful about our world." Chalmers is an atheist, but he says the simulation hypothesis has made him take the existence of god seriously.

Consider now Rizwan Virk's (2019) *The Simulation Hypothesis: An MIT Computer Scientist Shows Why AI, Quantum Physics and Eastern Mystics All Agree We Are in a Video Game*. This is a curious book. It was published by a company Virk started, which has published three books as of this writing, all by Virk. It draws on a physics/mysticism parallelism that has no critical foundation, as I demonstrate in great detail in Restivo (1983). And it is founded on the ill-conceived notion that quantum mechanics casts doubt on the reality of the material universe. For those of us who want to go on living, quantum mechanics does not cast doubt on the reality of crossing the street safely, obeying traffic lights, bandaging slight wounds, and not jumping out of airplanes without a parachute.

Why does the simulation hypothesis matter? Virk's answer is that we would increase our chances of surviving if we understood the nature of the video game we're in. How would we escape the simulation in order to do this? The standard arguments against the simulation hypothesis do not have the force of the profundity of the surface hypothesis, the science of crossing the street, to raise the spirit of Nietzsche. Physicist Lisa Randall, for example, wonders simply about why a "higher species" would want to bother putting us in a simulation. Once we understand that the brain is not an isolated system in our skulls, consciousness is not in the brain (see chapter 10), humans are radically social in evolutionary terms, and we can account for God sociologically (Restivo, 2021), the supports for BIV and simulation thinking collapse along, perhaps, with the supports for philosophy without stop signs.

The God in the Simulation

In his book on "virtual worlds," Chalmers (2022b: xx) almost immediately alerts us to the fact that God has a prominent role in this story; this is a journey on which we will encounter "time-hallowed philosophical questions such as 'Is there a God?'" The simulation hypothesis would be impossible without the provocation of deceptive demons, indeed "an all-powerful and all-deceiving God" (Chalmers, 2022b: 51). This is just another example of philosophy being driven by nonsense posing as reasoned argument about epistemology. Other instances of this sort of nonsense posing as reasoned discourse occur throughout the book, for example in Chalmers's (2022b: 121) discussion of evil demons and detectable and undetectable illusions. On page 165, we encounter "complex states of consciousness in God's mind." Why even mention this if there isn't some shred of evidence for such states? The reason has to be that philosophy is always traveling on roads without stop signs, like theologians who imagine that if you can imagine something it must be real or at least have some role to play in argumentation.

God shows up again in Chalmers's (2022b: 168–69) it-from-bit creation hypothesis, which "combines the it-from-bit hypothesis and the creation hypothesis . . . by saying that the physical world was created by a creator and is made of bits." He doesn't argue that the it-from-bit creation hypothesis and the simulation hypothesis are true; only that if you accept one you should accept the other: "These hypotheses are two ways of describing the same situation."

The it-from-bit hypothesis (Chalmers, 2022a) is a little bit like Wheeler's (1989) famous "it from bit" hypothesis that all of reality is grounded in information. Wheeler put that forward as a hypothesis about physics, that physics might be grounded in the interplay of information. But this was meant to be a hypothesis about reality. It wasn't one that made reality some kind of illusion. Physics is still real. It's grounded in information. If we are in a virtual reality, we're living in an "it from bit" universe where all this is grounded in information. Of course, that information might itself be grounded in processes in a computer in the next universe up. We'll have many levels of reality, but all of it is real.

Posthumans running a simulation are like gods. And those imagining these scenarios are prepared to posit a polytheism involving demigods at various levels of reality. All of the demigods except those at the fundamental level can be sanctioned by more powerful gods living at lower levels (Bostrom, 2003:12). These are the elements of a naturalistic theogony. We have to consider, Bostrom writes, the "real possibility" that our simulators will reward or punish us in an afterlife. And then he gives us a Pascal's wager. Faced with the fundamental uncertainty of simulators who can reward or punish, "even the basement civilization may have a reason to behave ethically." Through some recursive moral logic, we might arrive at a universal ethical imperative "which it would be in everybody's self-interest to obey, as it were 'from nowhere.'"

Chalmers has described the being responsible for this hyper-realistic simulation we may or may not be in as a "programmer in the next universe up," perhaps one we mortals might consider a god of some sort—though not necessarily in the traditional sense. It might be a teenage hacker running several universes in the background, but it might be someone all-knowing and all-powerful!

Let's consider Chalmers's ubiquitous use of the term "hypothesis." A hypothesis is a proposed preliminary explanation for a phenomenon. For a hypothesis to be a scientific hypothesis, the scientific perspective requires that there be an empirical rationale for it and that one can test it. Scientists generally base scientific hypotheses on previous observations that cannot satisfactorily be explained with the available scientific theories. Chalmers should stop using the term "hypothesis" and use something like "an idea that came to me," "an idle speculation," etc. Even "working hypothesis" would demand more of Chalmers than he can deliver. He seems to acknowledge this, as we will soon see.

On page 170 Chalmers introduces a series of propositions that begin with the words "Suppose God." What's the point of such a supposition if there is no God? By page 347, he is discussing simulation theodicy: "A theodicy is a theological explanation of why God might permit evil in the world. A simulation theodicy does the same for simulators." Why introduce theodicy and theology at all if they are scientifically irrelevant?

On pages 451 and following, Chalmers writes about Gods and evil demons. What he is trying to draw our attention to is that reasoning well can lead us to the truth: "When we reason well enough about mathematics to prove that two plus three is five, then we can know that two plus three is five." Chalmers has an enormous amount of faith in the individual's capacity to reason through to truths. This is the fallacy of the philosopher's conceit. It is based on the myth of individualism, the basic driving force behind classical philosophy, which can proceed without due attention to social interactions and social practice. We don't "reason" our way to $2 + 3 = 5$; we practice our way to that equality by way of interactions and communication in the everyday social world of accumulated and shared experiences.

If we have a simulator, it would not be worthy of worship. If the Abrahamic God exists, Chalmers would not consider him worthy of worship. He claims he is not religious; he is an atheist "open to the idea of a creator who is close to all-powerful, all-knowing, and all-good. I had once thought that this idea is inconsistent with a naturalistic view of the world, but the simulation idea makes it consistent. There remains a more fundamental reason for my atheism, however: I do not think any being is worthy of worship" (2022b: 144).

Chalmers (2022b: 73) does say early on that the "perfect simulation" hypothesis isn't a scientific hypothesis. We could not distinguish between a perfect simulation and an unsimulated world. This makes it difficult to imagine what evidence would count for or against the simulation hypothesis. Vienna Circle philosophers would then say the hypothesis is meaningless. Chalmers claims they are wrong. We may not have a scientific hypothesis, but it makes "perfect sense as a philosophical hypothesis about the nature of our world." Surely, Carnap and his colleagues would consider this utter nonsense. There are other grounds for dismissing Chalmers's "philosophical hypothesis." The very idea of philosophy loses its already-unsteady grip on reality in a world that has added sociology to the core sciences of physics, chemistry, biology, psychology, and economics.

One of my interlocutors suggested that AI researchers will want to know why we can't just attach a brain to a robotic body. If the question is about an artificial brain, we can basically do that now. Autonomous robots' brains are technological composites of laser scanners, cameras, radar, lidar, microphones, force-torque sensors, spectrometers, infrared and ultrasound sensors, and image-recognition software. Such robots, like autonomous cars, often need human "backups." But the question is really a BIV question. The robot is the vat. The brain could either be a fleshy brain grown in a petri dish or a human brain "taken" from a deceased or living human. The petri dish brain in a robot is pretty much a science fiction scenario, but not entirely. Scientists have created neuronal media that support the basic synaptic functions and activity of human neurons; live brain cells from patients can be grown and aged in a petri dish. Biological cells have been used to create small clusters of neurons. And a team of scientists in Düsseldorf, Germany, has grown mini brains in petri dishes that have developed organic structures resembling eyes. But the key question my interlocutor had in mind was: Could a functioning human brain "taken" from a deceased human be attached to a robot and continue to function as it did in the living human with all of its memories and sensory connections to the robot's body intact? The answer is no because, as my model demonstrates, the working living human brain is a complex network of networks informationally linked to a body and environment. Removing the brain from a human, assuming it could be kept "alive," would destroy those links and information flows.

CONCLUSION

There are good reasons we humans should be fearful in some fundamental way. We are, for all of our technologies and literary and scientific achievements, strangers in a strange world. We are not constructed in a way that would allow us to grasp the nature, scope, and scale of the universe we have so cleverly discovered and explored. I don't know that this fear can be conquered, but I think it can be tamed. We can learn to leave childish things behind. We can learn to live without gods and an afterlife. If we cultivate this way of life and a sociological imagination, we should be able to live our lives without worrying about evil demons, without being tormented by whether we are Zhuang Zhou or a butterfly. We are a fragile species and we're not very good at leaving childish things behind. But some of us do seem to know that however strange and counter-intuitive quantum mechanics seems to be, it is incidental at best to the profundity of the surface.

Chapter 9

Robots, AI, Brains, and Bodies in the Information Age

Experiments in robotics and artificial intelligence (AI) are blurring the boundary between the living and dead (perhaps one source of the zombianism that is so prominent in popular culture). We need to consider more critically what is at stake in the development of socially intelligent, sociable, and emotional robots. Perhaps we may have to learn to respect the new emerging material lifeworld that we are creating in our own image. The Kasparov–Deep Blue chess match was billed as a "man versus machine" event and reinforced predictions about the emergence of machines with emotions.

Let's consider the Kasparov–Deep Blue match. The rhetoric of "man versus machine" masked the fact that Kasparov and Deep Blue were stand-ins for two networks of humans (including experts on chess and computers) and machines. "Man" is already a cog in a cyborg network. As for machines with emotions and consciousness, the problem resolves itself differently if we proceed from the idea of "robots 'r' us," which gives us a new life form, or if we think of "robots as robots" which gives us machines; and of course, there is a middle ground, the Technium, an idea we owe to Kevin Kelly (2012). The Technium is the self-organized global network of interlocked technologies; it is not alive, but it exhibits lifelike behaviors. It is the "inevitable" next stage in the process that gave us self-organized life.

The "robots 'r' us" position leads to skepticism about whether robots could ever be conscious in the way that we are conscious or experience emotions in the ways that we humans do. If we adopt the "robots as robots" position, we are encouraged to think in terms of machine consciousness and machine emotions. It's important to remember that we humans are organic machines, so we already know that machines can be conscious and feel. It might then be possible for inorganic machines to develop their own forms of consciousness and emotions. The Technium concept suggests, on the one hand, hybrid machines and, on the other, sociologically impoverished futures. I am not dismissing the concept of the Technium here, only asking that it be less a technological fix than a concept that signifies a profound integration of the organic, the inorganic, and the social. In all of these cases, robotics engineers and futurists are going to have to pay more attention to (1) the role of mimesis and rhythmicity in the evolution of human communication, consciousness, and emotions; and (2) the nature of interaction rituals and interaction ritual chains and their significance for the emergence of consciousness and emotions. The technological materialization of mimesis, rhythm, and entrainment may be sufficient to generate embryonic awareness and proto-consciousness in near-future robots.

We can now see the significance of dancing and why robots should be able to dance, something I pointed out in 2005. Dance, as I pointed out earlier (chapter 5), is the coarse expression of the fine-grained rhythmicity that is innate to all levels of life, from cells to bodies; and even social systems have their rhythms, even societies and groups dance. If we want to build robots that are conscious and emotional, we will have to teach them to dance and build rhythm into their silicon and steel. There is, in fact, a movement in robotics that recognizes the importance of dance without yet connecting it to consciousness and emotions (Heimerdinger and LaViers, 2019; LaViers et al., 2011, 2018; Marino, et al., 2016).

The work on social and sociable robots and affective computing has created a social space of border tensions between minds, brains, bodies, machines, and humans, and scientific and theologico-religious authority. Not only are we reinventing bodies, we are reinventing science and posing new challenges to religion and ethics. As a species, we are working globally on so many different planes of action that we are faced with the unintended, unpredictable, and unknowable consequences of a multiplicity of multiplier effects. I am not worried as some are about "post-human" futures, about human beings being "replaced" by machines. Sooner or later, we are going to be replaced by something (or nothingness); that shouldn't be the issue. The more immediate issue is: What will happen to us if more and more of us spend increasing amounts of time with robots capable of becoming Mr. Rogers or Kate Smith and incapable of becoming Nietzsche or Virginia Woolf?

Social Versus Sociable Robots

The term "social robot" is used in at least two ways. It can mean (1) robots that socially interact with humans, and (2) collective robots inspired by social animals. A "social robot" is a robot designed for social interaction with humans and in principle—in the short or long run—capable of expressing emotions, demonstrating consciousness, and thinking and moving about autonomously (Restivo, 2001; Restivo and Steinhauer, 2000). More than this, such a robot would be able to move rhythmically in conversations, both in terms of speech and in terms of body. Such robots would be important in two ways. First, they would represent a significant addition to the forms of companionship available to us. Second, they could be used in experiments testing fundamental ideas in the social theory of mind. The more "social" the robot, the more humanoid it would be. This could actually obstruct using them in experiments because they would be "too humanlike." In this regard, then, the term "sociable robot" is not appropriate.

"Sociable" in ordinary dictionary terms means "fond of company" or "characterized by friendly companionship." Cynthia Breazeal (2002: 1), an MIT robotics engineer who has pioneered sociable robot engineering, describes a sociable robot as a robot capable of communicating, interacting, understanding, and relating to us in personal ways. Ideally, such robots would be capable of reciprocal self-understanding and empathy with humans: "In short, a sociable robot is socially intelligent in a human-like way and interacting with it is like interacting with another person. At the pinnacle of achievement, they could befriend us, as we could them." Breazeal goes on to point out that science fiction has demonstrated how such technologies "could enhance our lives and benefit society."

There are, however, cautionary tales. Breazeal refers, for example, to Philip K. Dick's (1990) *Do Androids Dream of Electric Sheep*, which raises issues about approaching dreams of robots (sociable or otherwise) responsibly and ethically. Cute and adorable robots like Kismet, Breazeal's MIT PhD project, interestingly enough, provoked worried reactions when they came to public attention (e.g., Nightline, 2002). I also have some evidence from unpublished exploratory studies of similarly worried and cautious reactions to My Real Baby by children and adults. My Real Baby is an animatronic doll invented by MIT robotics engineer Rodney Brooks and originally manufactured in 1998 by his company, iRobot, in collaboration with Hasbro. One of my questions is then what is the counter-reaction to such views by sociable robotics engineers?

Engineering sociable robots programs out differences that make us (or at least the robot engineers) uncomfortable. Social robots, by contrast, could become Virginia Woolf or Oscar Wilde—or Al Capone. Social robots could develop cognitive and physical illnesses, disabilities, and various sorts of impairments.

Information technologies are ready targets for social criticism and critical theory, and for ethical analyses. Information itself has until recently escaped these critical and analytical tools (but see Roszak, 1986). The Critical Art Ensemble collective draws attention to the theological rhetoric that surrounds the human genome project and how it masks the eugenic origins of this discourse. Genesis creator Eduardo Kac has tried to represent the continuity between imperialist ideology and reductionist genetics. He accomplishes this artistically by translating a passage from the King James Bible into Morse code and then translating the Morse code into a gene.

What is at stake here? Transgenic artists such as Kac may be creating early warning systems to alert us to the consequences of the world(s) we are fashioning for "nature," species, culture, and self in their independent and networked forms. The quotes around "nature" signal an increasing awareness that the very idea of nature is not as transparent, unified, or universal as we once assumed. Indeed, that signals that we should probably put quotation marks around all of the forms I listed with nature. We need to become comfortable with the idea of natures, just as we are learning to become more or less comfortable with the idea of sciences instead of Science and bodies instead of Body (and so selves instead of Self—"I am multitudes," Walt Whitman wrote). We are moving toward a pluralization of all of our basic categories and classification.

Living in Liminal Times

These are liminal times. Perhaps all times—or recurring moments in history—are liminal in some way. When I say "our time" is liminal, here in the early decades of the twenty-first century, I do so in recognition of a radical flux of categories, classifications, and cultural configurations local, regional, and global unlike anything we have ever seen or experienced. The categories, classifications, and configurations at issue at this juncture of history, culture, and biographies are fundamental. They represent the foundations of the world's cultures, values, norms, interests, and goals. Social movements and social changes in general have made such primordial classifications as male-female, life-death, nature-society, human-machine, person-fetus, and the classifications of sex and gender problematic. I don't mean to ignore earlier examples of this sort of problematic but rather to suggest that we are engaging a fundamentally qualitatively and quantitatively different problematic. The very idea of science has become problematic in three ways: (1) science and cultural studies have led us to a more complex social and cultural understanding of the sciences and the good terms associated with it: truth, objectivity, mathematics, logic, and reason; (2) the related engagement of Western modes of science with non-Western modes of thought and philosophy; and (3) the challenge of fake news, fake science, pseudo-science, and the triumph of media-driven opinions over evidence-based truths (on the post-truth society, see Restivo, 2022: 325–42).

Dichotomous and hierarchical thinking across the spectra of intellectual life have given way to thinking in terms of complexities, non-linearities, chaos, fractals, multiple logics, heterarchies, and networks. One of the characteristics of our liminal era is the proliferation of hybrid and monstrous entities and ideas. We are everywhere, in and out of the academy, in and out of the business community, in and out of all of our institutions, accosted by inter-, multi-, and transdisciplinarities. Competing theorists are charged with exploring new ways of organizing our categories and classifications and producing new ways of ordering the world that work under our new and radically changing circumstances. These efforts will in general and inevitably strike us as awkward, counter-intuitive, obscure, and even monstrous, but they draw our attention to the need to reconfigure, reconstitute, reform, revalue, and revolutionize our reigning categories and classifications.

Sociology itself may have to be reconfigured, and I will show what direction this might take in my final chapter. Sociology can be transformed without succumbing to the "end of the social" movement. One of the leaders of that movement, Bruno Latour, has tried to "reform" sociology without understanding first what it is that sociologists do and then ignoring the very nature of what science is and what a social science is and could be. There is no doubt that, as an intellectual industry, he has attracted an enormous amount of attention by being (above all else) an ideological entrepreneur and presenting his messages in the languages and rhetorics of theology, philosophy, and metaphysics. Our intellectual elites and public intellectuals are more comfortable with these languages and rhetorics than they are with the language and rhetoric of the social sciences. Those sciences are viewed as less robust than the physical and natural sciences, even though they have unrecognized levels of robustness and scientific integrity (see Restivo, 2017, 2018; and Collins, 1973, 1998). Intellectuals, journalists, and science watchers in general miss this because they are sociologically myopic and suffer from dissocism, the inability to "see" the social and to see it as a nexus of causes. Latour's efforts to develop an alternative to the constituting and constructive activities of social relations have failed because he is at heart anti-scientific (or better, non-scientific), reflecting his allegiance to ethnomethodology; non-evidentiary philosophy, theology, and metaphysics; and the cult of individualism (Restivo, 2011).

The traditional world of brains, minds, and bodies can no longer support our experiences and experiments. We need to think about things—ourselves above all—in new ways not grounded in categories, classifications, and configuration that have reigned for hundreds of years and in some cases for millennia. This has already taken root within the inner sanctum of the neurosciences (see Brothers, 1997; Donald, 2001; and Rose, 2005) and among at least some postmodernists in the humanities and social sciences.

Some of us have become frustrated with how resistant the body is to being disciplined. How should we address the regulatory norms through which the body is materialized? Notice that pluralization and disciplining impose new restraints and regulations on bodies and simultaneously provoke multiple forms of bodies. As I noted earlier, we now have a public space of reconfiguring bodies and selves, a space marked by transgendered and transexed bodies, LGBTQ+, homo-, hetero-, and trans-normative relationships. Will we find our future in Marx's realm of freedom, Kelly's Technium, the Matrix, or Armageddon?

CONCLUSION

When I (as a social scientist) say that humans are social, I mean that they are constructed out of social interactions, that they are social structures. I also mean that their social nature must be constantly reinforced through social interactions. What we experience and conceive of as individuals are from this perspective networks of social relationships. This is a given, whether we are sociable or sociopaths, likeable or not, normal or deviant. To be human means to have potentials for conflictful as well as cooperative relationships, contentious as well as companionable relationships, and the potential to make mistakes. In constructing sociable robots, especially those based on the more psychologically grounded social theories, robotics engineers seem to be driven to program out aspects of being human that for one reason or another they don't like or that make them personally uncomfortable. Such robots might eventually have a place in our society, but they will not be social robots. Kismet could become Mr. or Mrs. Rogers, but Kismet could never become Nietzsche or Virginia Woolf.

It is a short step to recognizing that not much—or perhaps not enough—is being done that acknowledges potential unintended consequences in this field. We should be working up models and scenarios that explore unintended consequences. Articulating unintended consequences in a sense violates the principle of unintended consequences, but once we bring the principle into our sights, it will not be too difficult to play out some hypothetical stories. In this way, we may be able to lower the probabilities for the more disastrous unintended consequences to become actualized, even if we cannot in principle avoid all such outcomes.

Social robots should be distinguished from other socially interactive systems (e.g., software agents, swarms, distributed and collective intelligences). The mark of a social robot should be its capacity for rhythmic entrainment with the humans (and robots) it is interacting with. It should have many if not all of the characteristics Breazeal (2002: 229–42) outlines in her grand challenges (e.g., embodied discourse), but in the end it must be able to participate in interaction rituals and ritual chains. Without the possibility of building robots capable of participating in the rituals of everyday life robotics engineers will fall short of their most ambitious visions in this field. Their robots will be little more than coded complexes of mimicry, little more than toys with chips.

We can look forward to robots in "just like us" terms, robots with human forms of mentalities and emotions, or to robots in "robots as robots" terms, robots with machine mentalities and emotions, or perhaps to hybrid robots, who possess hybrid mentalities and emotions. In any case, humans are going to be the "likeness" against which we measure the qualities and achievements of the "Others" in our midst. Social robots in our midst will confront us with questions of what alternative forms of embodiment and semio-materiality mean for us as humans, as men, women, and children of culture, ethnicity, class, sex, gender, and age. Sociable robots will be our new Other companions, taking the places of or joining our dogs, cats, and human caretakers.

Who are these robots for? Are they for all of us or just some of us? Are they for us as persons or just for some parts of us? What and who are and will they be good for? Will they come into the world as appliances or humanoids, treated the way we treat our stoves and refrigerators in the former case, or treated as partners in love, sex, companionship, and friendship in the latter case? Will they give us a new class of industrial robots or a new class of robots with feelings and self-awareness that will be enslaved for scientific experiments, work, warfare, and sex? There are invidious implications in these sorts of questions. I have no doubt on the positive side that social and sociable robots will help us understand our dynamic and social selves, bodies, and social groups. They will problematize our embodiment, our senses, our sensuo-erotics. And as these robots come into the world we will come into the world differently, and we will matter differently. Social, sociable, and Other robots should be understood in the context of specific and overlapping social locations and not simply in terms of the ideas and practices of individual scientists and engineers.

Attention to social locations means, more broadly, attention to historical, cultural, and social locations locally, regionally, and globally. In the end, the limits of robots of all forms are not in the limits of silicon and steel but in the limits of our interpretative courage and technological recklessness. We really have no more and nothing different to fear from robots than we do from each other. When we meet these robots, we will meet ourselves.

Social, sociable, and Other robotics are important vectors in the movement of science and technology across the world. This movement is a multilinear, multicultural dialectic that heralds the creation/emergence of a new form(s) of social order. The story of this social order begins: "In the beginning was *information*." And perhaps this social order will intersect with a new evolutionary order, *the Technium*, or some new order of bio-social-technological entities, *The Cyborgs*.

Chapter 10

The Sociology of Consciousness

I have remarked on the "hard problem" of consciousness throughout the previous chapters. In this chapter, I want to bring my scattered remarks together and contextualize them. I have alluded in various ways to a sociological answer to the hard problem of consciousness. Is it possible to construct a sociologically coherent theory of consciousness? Without a way of grounding consciousness in the social world, we become trapped in the "hard problem." Let's collect the basic elements of what I've said so far about consciousness. First, I've argued that the wrong scientists using the wrong tools have been looking in the wrong place for consciousness. Second, I've argued that if we turn to sociology and draw on its tools, methods, and theories we will be guided to look for consciousness in the social world and not *in* the brain. The same is true if we turn to anthropology. My degrees are in sociology, but all of my mentors have been credentialed anthropologists or sociologist ethnographers. Therefore, I don't recognize a distinction between the two disciplines in my education or my research. Following the sociology/anthropology trail, we will also be able to avoid dualist thinking and the "God" problem. I've offered some preliminary ideas that associate consciousness with rhythmicity in social relations and considered the possibility that we are dealing with a relational and perhaps field phenomenon. Let's now start from the beginning and consider history and context.

PRIMITIVE SELF-AWARENESS

The problem of consciousness has in roots in our primitive self-awareness. This gives rise to a vocabulary of mind, thought, imagination, cognition, experience, and perception. Some level of cultural and linguistic evolution must be reached before humans begin to experience a transparent introspection. This unfolds, notably in philosophical circles, into a sense that we are on the one hand simply aware, on the other that we are aware of being aware, and then that there might be levels and orders of consciousness. Philosophers and theologians have struggled to make sense of awareness phenomena since ancient times. The problem and the concept of "consciousness" begins to take some scientific shape in the works of Western philosophers from the time of Descartes and Locke onward. From that point onward it rapidly becomes a boundary object (Star and Griesemer, 1989: 393). Boundary objects are characterized by a plasticity that allows them to be used across various disciplines and at the same time a certain robustness that allows them to maintain an identity in the various disciplines and sites of use: "They are weakly structured in common use and become strongly structured in individual-site use. They may be abstract or concrete. They have different meanings in different social worlds but their structure is common enough to more than one world to make them recognizable, a means of translation. The creation and management of boundary objects is key in developing and maintaining coherence across intersecting social worlds." The degree of coherence is more assumed than real given the variety of disciplinary uses and languages they are subject to. Consciousness has been claimed as a proper subject for philosophy, theology, psychology, linguistics, biology, physics, neuroscience, and so on. Sociologists and anthropologists have not been very visible in the arena of consciousness studies, but it has not escaped their attention (e.g., Cohen and Rapport, 1995; Whitehead, 2008).

There is an interesting etymological feature of the concept of "consciousness" from a sociological perspective. Dating from the sixteenth century, the word "conscious" was derived from the Latin "conscius," "con" meaning "together" and "scio" meaning "to know." In this sense, consciousness meant "having joint or common knowledge with another" (Lewis, 1990: Chapter 8). I will pass over the history of the confused association of "conscious" and "conscience."

Defining Consciousness

It will be worthwhile at this point to consider common usage and philosophical usage. Common dictionary definitions identify consciousness as a state of awareness, an awareness or perception of something in the mind and in the world. Philosophers have tried to pin down the concept which comes up in their studies of knowledge, intentionality, introspection, and phenomenal experience. The result of their efforts from Descartes and Locke on have not been at all satisfying. Stuart Sutherland (1989: 95) has described it as "a fascinating but elusive phenomenon. It is impossible to specify what it is, what it does, or why it evolved. Nothing worth reading has been written on it." We are enmeshed in a wide range of experiences involving awareness that knot up the problem of consciousness. There seems to be little reason to question a basic level of awareness in humans. But if awareness of our surroundings is the root of our concept of consciousness, this opens up the possibility of consciousness being a feature of even the simplest animal life. If awareness of awareness is our criterion, this seems to favor its restriction to humans who have matured past infancy. It is hard to get beyond our intuitive sense of consciousness, even if we are philosophers. Ryle (1949), as we saw earlier, proposed to unknot the concept by making it (mind and consciousness) one with our understanding of behavior and language. This had the advantage of avoiding the tendency of consciousness studies to devolve into some form of dualism.

One of the suggestions for sorting out the difficulties with the concept of consciousness was to distinguish P-consciousness from A-consciousness—that is, respectively, phenomenal consciousness from access consciousness (Block, 1998). This distinction did not lead to consensus among philosophers about the nature and function of consciousness. In fact, it led Lycan (1996: 1–4) to propose eight distinct types of consciousness. Philosophers have offered many reasons to criticize Descartes's dualism, but various forms of monism have not been able to garner a consensus. The Newtonian tradition in science has led some philosophers to assume that there must be a purely physical solution to the hard problem of consciousness. Neuroscientists have constructed neural theories; physicists have favored quantum solutions (e.g., Penrose, 1989; Penrose and Hameroff, 1995) and relativistic theories (e.g., Lahav and Neemeh, 2022). The contemporary situation seems to favor a Rylean solution rather than exotic quantum and relativity notions or totally neuronal theories. One could say about consciousness what Voltaire said about love, that the term is given to a thousand chimera. All that can be said at this point is that no one has come up with a universally acceptable solution to the hard problem of consciousness, or even one that commands the allegiance of a significant proportion of the scientific community. The reason for this, in my view, is that the wrong scientists using the wrong tools, methods, and theories have been looking for it in the wrong places. Ryle has given us the most philosophically sound solution to the hard problem, but there is something unsatisfying about his solution because it does not address the individual experience of awareness, of awareness of awareness, of "something" going on in "the head." Let's turn now to what light sociology and anthropology might be able to throw on the problem.

Can Social Science Solve the
Hard Problem of Consciousness?

One of the first provocations that set me on the road to a sociological perspective on consciousness and the social brain was Nietzsche's (1887/1974:

298–99, aphorism 354) remark that "Consciousness is really only a net of communication [*Verbindungsnetz*] between human beings; it is only as such that it had to develop; a solitary human being who lived like a beast of prey would not have needed it. . . . Consciousness does not really belong to man's individual existence but rather to his social or herd nature." The social science of this insight begins to crystallize in the works of the early social psychologists and social philosophers and notably in the works of G. H. Mead (1934: 18). Mead found no evidence for Darwin's notion of consciousness as independent of the mutual behavioral adjustment of organisms. Instead, Mead argued, we are forced to understand consciousness as emerging from such behavior: "far from being a precondition of the social act, the social act is the precondition of it."

C. Wright Mills (1939) argued that Mead's theories of mind and consciousness had not been exploited by sociologists. Fifty years later, Randall Collins (1989) could still argue that these materials were underdeveloped. This failure was underlined by the publication of a social theory of mind influenced by Mead's work written not by a sociologist but by psychiatrist and neuroscientist Leslie Brothers (1997). Brothers is widely recognized for introducing the modern idea of the social brain in a 1990 article. The late twentieth and early twentieth centuries witnessed an impressive growth of literature in the neuro-, life, and social sciences exploring the social aspects of brain, mind, and consciousness. This literature formed the foundation of my research, writing, and lecturing on these topics beginning in the 1990s. My remarks on the social nature of consciousness in the previous chapters reflect my efforts to shape these developments into a coherent sociology of consciousness.

Consciousness in Sociological Perspective

Let's collect my earlier claims about consciousness:

1. Consciousness represents the living shape of our community.
2. Consciousness is an expression of our existence as social beings.
3. Face-to-face relationships are the basic means for the emergence of consciousness, mind, and emotions.
4. Consciousness and emotions are relational; they are in-between phenomena and not phenomena that are generated and sustained within the individual or the individual brain.
5. Rhythmic entrainment engenders a field (see below on the field concept) that carries emotional communication and consciousness. Introducing the idea of a field here is a working conjecture that does not have a strong empirical rationale but can be grounded in research.

6. Consciousness is a by-product of the innate rhythmicity of humans. It is our capacity for dance as an in-between conduit that generates consciousness.
7. Consciousness arises as a consequence of coordinated activities generating rhythmic entrainment and resonance.

If we consider these statements proto-hypotheses, then what is the rationale that grounds them? The underlying rationale for these proto-hypotheses is the fact that we humans are always, already, and everywhere social. Basic awareness does not emerge in individuals, but in the awareness that others are aware. If Descartes had understood this he would have written "*cogitamus ergo sumus*," not "*cogito ergo sum*." An even stronger sociological imagination would have had him reverse the *cogito* to "*sumus ergo cogitamus*" (Whitehead, 2008: 11). That degree of sociological imagination was born with Durkheim's insights into the significance of shared experiences and their relation to contagion and empathy (and see Frith, 2008; and on sympathetic engagement, see Trevarthen, 1979). This is an evolved adaptation that allows humans to share their collective representations of the world: "Collective representations can have well-defined cortical representations" (Whitehead, 2008: 55; and see pp. 43–121 on "The Social Brain" with contributions by Turner and Whitehead; Chiao, Li, and Harrada; Sinigaglia; and Whitehead). The anthropologist Bruce Kapferer (1995: 134) demonstrates the alignment of anthropology with this social perspective. Consciousness, he writes, is always embodied, always "constituted and expressed through the action of the body." But it is formed "through its engagement with other human beings in the world." This blossoming research frontier that emerged in the 1990s demonstrated, among other things relevant to my consciousness proposals, that emotions appeared to be post-construals after behaviors were already underway. This is remindful of Libet's famous experiment. Libet (1985) demonstrated that the unconscious electrical processes in the brain called readiness potential precede conscious decisions to perform volitional, spontaneous acts. This implied that unconscious neuronal processes precede volitional acts. We experience these acts as self-willed. Readiness potential was discovered by Kornhuber and Deecke (1965). The experiment has been immersed in controversy because it undermined the idea that we have free will and because of its implicit assumptions (Rigoni et al., 2011).

Increasingly, researchers were becoming aware of the pervasive influence of culture on brain anatomy and of the brain as a "doing organ" rather than a "thinking organ" (Brown, 1991; and for an early insight into these issues see Benn, 1972; and Turner, R., 2002). The complexity of my social network social brain model reflects the growing recognition of the complexity of emotions and consciousness (Cardenia, 2008).

The multilevel nature of emotions is intimately related to the multilevel phenomenon of consciousness. This system is reflected in different forms of connectedness within and outside of the individual. This suggests a multilevel embedded-systems approach to understanding and mapping emotions and consciousness in the social brain-in-culture-in-the-world, "an equivalent of a kind of entanglement of activity in individual brains" (Combs and Krippner, 2008: 273). Connolly (2002: 7, 10, 13) expresses a similar understanding of this complexity in his notion of the layered nature of thinking and culture. This sort of theorizing supports a resonance theory and the idea that behavioral synchronicity is coupled to neural synchronicity.

The Field Concept

The most controversial feature in my proposal for a sociology of consciousness is the concept of a *field*, which I assume is generated when two or more human beings come into mutual presence. I assume that the resonating humans in mutual presence generate a field in a way that is a form of mutual inductance. The field is the medium across which emotions, consciousness, and communication travel. Is there any natural mechanism that could account for such a field? Scientists have identified central oscillators in brain circuits that generate rhythmic firing patterns that regulate many bodily functions. MIT neuroscientists Takatoh, Prevosto, et al. (2022; and see Dominiak et al., 2019) recently discovered the neuronal identity and mechanism of the whisking oscillator in mice, the oscillator that controls the synchronous rhythmic sweeping of tactile whiskers in mice.

In other research related to rhythmicity, synchronicity, and field generation, Wikström et al. (2022) have discovered inter-brain synchronization without physical co-presence during cooperative online gaming. They point out that inter-brain synchronization during social interaction has been linked to closeness and cooperation. Their study goes beyond this to demonstrate synchronization without physical co-presence but during a collaborative coordinated task. Another potential source of the field I hypothesize to be activated by co-presence is the magnetic forces associated with every cell in our bodies. Magnetic fields affect our biological systems to various degrees. Pribram proposed that the heart and body generate low-frequency oscillations—afferent neural, hormonal, and electrical patterns that can carry emotional information—and high-frequency oscillations that can carry consciousness. It is hypothetically possible that these rhythmic patterns can be transmitted into the environment and be detected by others (McCraty, 2015, including references to Pribram's and related work in an extensive bibliography).

CONCLUSION

There has been a sociology and anthropology of the brain and consciousness since the earliest days of the development of these fields. Durkheim, Marx, Nietzsche, Charlotte Perkins Gilman, and others theorized and speculated on the social nature of consciousness, emotions, and the brain. The beginnings of a sophisticated sociological theory of consciousness crystallized in the works of G. H. Mead. There was little in the way of cumulative scholarship in this area following Mead, but the threads of his work were picked up by C. Wright Mills, Randall Collins, Charles Whitehead, Anthony Cohen, and Nigel Rapport, myself, and others. This literature, already small to begin with, was completely overshadowed by the works of philosophers, psychologists, and others. Those others struggled with the "hard problem" of consciousness, and in spite of a millennia-long discourse, little headway was made in achieving a consensus on the very nature of consciousness, let alone any explanatory approach that could mobilize widespread support. The problem all along has been the influence of the myth of individualism, dissocism, the fallacy of introspective transparency, and an understanding of the brain as an independent biomedical organ that was supposed to be the font of all of our behaviors, thoughts, and emotions; it was the assumed location of mind and consciousness. The bold move of the sociologists and anthropologists was to eliminate the myth of individualism and brain-centric, brain-in-a-vat thinking. This freed them to work toward a viable, grounded sociological theory of consciousness, emotions, and the brain. That relatively small, virtually invisible research arena has given me the resources to pursue a synthesis leading to a model of the social brain.

Chapter 11

The Social Life of the Brain

THE SOCIAL BRAIN EMERGES

Challenges to the concept of the brain as an independent, isolated biological organ began to appear in the 1950s. Students of primate behavior had been exploring a possible relationship between brain size and the size and complexity of social groups. They eventually proposed the social intelligence hypothesis. Social intelligence, it appeared, was the driving force in the increasing size of the human brain. In other words, larger brains were needed to deal with the increasing complexity of human societies. It now became important to tease this hypothesis and explore whether bigger brains were driving the increasing complexity of societies, or increasing complexity was driving bigger brains. The most plausible alternative was that the brain and society were coupled in co-evolution. This theorizing slowly evolved into a social brain hypothesis.

Originally the social brain was identified with specific regions of the brain (such as the amygdala and the insula). As research in this field has progressed it has become increasingly clear that the brain is a complex organ that originates and functions at the nexus of biological, environmental, and social forces. The whole brain is shaped by these forces. By the 2000s, the social brain hypothesis was finding its way into studies of autism, schizophrenia, and other classic topics in psychiatry. Even within the field of fMRI research a growing body of evidence shows that brain processes, and complex processes in particular, aren't limited to small parts of the brain. The brain is complex and networked and "zooming out" in fMRI studies is demonstrating this (e.g., Noble, et al., 2022).

THE NEUROSCIENCE REVOLUTION

The neuroscience revolution of the late twentieth century provoked a brain-self-help book industry. That industry was fueled by traditional ideas about the brain as an independent biological entity and the ideology of the independent individual. Colorful brain scans pinpointing the "brain at work" fueled the public imagination and support for the neurosciences. In the 1990s and early 2000s brain research initiatives were proclaimed by governments around the world. These initiatives were founded on the assumption that the brain was the causal font of all of our behaviors, emotions, and thoughts. This assumption is stated specifically in Bush's 1990 Decade of the Brain proclamation and in Obama's 2013 BRAIN initiative. During that same period, a new brain paradigm emerged along with a surge of research around the concepts of enhanced environments, epigenetics, neuroplasticity, and mirror neurons. That new paradigm was the *social* brain. We are now seeing self-help books that are based on some version of a social brain paradigm.[1]

The social brain paradigm will eventually supersede all conventional thinking that makes the brain the originating locus of all of our thoughts, emotions, and behaviors. The social brain model I introduce in this chapter is an innovative undertaking, but it is not so much "new" as it is an effort to integrate and extrapolate the various emerging proposals designed to revise classical thinking about the brain/mind/body and the directions such revisions should be taking. This integration has led to the most highly networked model of the brain in the brain-in-the-world literature.

Hierarchical models have dominated approaches to the modern understanding of cognition and consciousness for most of the last two centuries and longer. Hierarchical thinking guided model and theory building across the entire spectrum of the sciences during most of this time. During the second half of the twentieth century, postmodernist thinkers led or provoked the struggle against classical philosophy and psychology. This struggle undermined categories and classifications that had reigned for millennia in some cases and for hundreds of years in others. Male and female, life and death, nature and nurture are among the most prominent of the dichotomies that have fractured along with the brain/mind/body trichotomy.

The world of models and theories has increasingly come to be dominated by complexity, non-linearity, fractals, chaos, and multiple logical systems. Hierarchies and dichotomies have been abandoned in favor of networks which are better suited to the complexities and connectivities we have begun to encounter in our search for causes and consequences across the sciences. Postmodernists often seemed to be on the edge of or falling into the abyss of nihilism, a false anarchism of "anything goes," or the trap of naïve relativism.

On the positive side, they provided insights on how to realistically revise our ideas about truth, objectivity, and science. Most importantly, they helped direct our attention to the social and cultural causes and contexts of our thoughts, emotions, and behaviors. Network thinking has helped to transform the way we understand the brain. The networked social brain is the topic of this chapter. I begin with the story of how we arrived at current models of the networked brain.

The Social Intelligence Hypothesis

Our story begins with the social intelligence hypothesis. To review, this hypothesis was designed to explain the size of human brains. The idea was that increasingly complex and dense social interactions were the driving forces behind the large brains of *Homo sapiens*. Around two million years ago the brain more than doubled in size. This was correlated with the fact that humans were living in larger and larger and more and more complex groups. It was assumed that a larger brain reflected the need for a larger mental capacity to keep track of people and relationships in social groups that were growing in size.

A second period of growth in the brain occurred between six hundred thousand and two hundred thousand years ago. This period of growth was thought to be most likely related to cultural growth and especially to the evolution of language. However, the human brain experienced a decrease in size about three thousand years ago (DeSilva et al., 2021). One plausible explanation for this change is that the brain became smaller as a consequence of the expansion of cognition into the society at large. More and more of the weight of information and knowledge was being carried outside the human brain per se.

Social intelligence was considered a critical factor in brain growth. The social intelligence hypothesis evolved into the social brain hypothesis. This development was based on research that showed that primates have unusually large brains for their body size among the vertebrates. The explanation takes off from the social intelligence hypothesis; larger brains evolved to cope with increasingly complex social systems. In fact, the general hypothesis, applied to all vertebrates, is that brain size is correlated with social complexity. It was initially hypothesized that primates evolved large brains to manage their unusually complex social systems. This hypothesis, originally applied in an evolutionary context to all vertebrate taxa, has been modified based on research that shows social brain differences in (using the classical distinctions) non-anthropoid primates, anthropoids, and other mammals. Brain size varies monotonically as a function of group size in primates. Functions are known as monotonic if they are increasing or decreasing along their entire domain.

In other mammals and birds the relationship is qualitative. Larger brains are associated with differences in mating systems, in particular with pair-bonding. Researchers are uncertain about the reason for this association. We know that the anthropoid primates appear to have generalized pair-bonded mating to other non-reproductive relationships (e.g., "friendships"). What is at issue is why bonded relationships are so cognitively demanding that they require larger brains. This issue can be addressed by considering that social life in humans is not based on pair-bonding dyads but rather on social triads. Larger brains are associated with increasingly complex and dense social networks based on the triad as the fundamental unit of analysis. It does not seem likely that there is a single causal pathway from brain size to social complexity or social complexity to brain size. Co-evolution is the most plausible way to view the relationship between brain and society.

The Social Brain Hypothesis

Leslie Brothers is widely credited with introducing the concept of the social brain to the neuroscience community in 1990. Brothers was well placed to make this introduction. She is not only a psychiatrist and neuroscientist but rare among her colleagues in her command of the sociological imagination. The model she introduced involves neural regions rather than the brain as a whole. The significance of her model is that it shifted the long-standing view of the brain as a biological entity essentially independent of social and cultural influences to a social entity. The traditional theories of brain and mind supported and were grounded in the myth of individualism. Brothers based her model on social brain research among non-human primates that came into prominence in the 1950s and thereafter. The increasing attention to the links between social complexity, social intelligence, and brain size fueled the social brain concept that Brothers finally crystallized in her 1990 paper.

How does a regional theory of the social brain work? It begins by asking the question: How do we infer the mental states of others? If we suppose that this ability is based on simulation and empathy, then (relying on a more or less traditional view of localization of brain functions) we can identify this ability with the premotor cortex and the insula. If we assume a more organized theory of mind, then we are pointed to the medial prefrontal cortex and the temporo-parietal junction, among other regions. The orbitofrontal cortex, a region in the frontal lobes, is associated with processing rewards. Lesions in this area are associated with severe disruptions in social behavior. At the same time cognition in other regions remains relatively intact. The insula, located underneath the frontal cortex, represents bodily states such as pain and empathy; it is active when we become aware of the pain of others. The brain regions involved in social cognition are sensitive to context, and their activation is modulated by social context and volitional regulation. All of this still leaves us with the mystery of explaining how inference works. The primates all show precursors to inference, but it is most highly developed in humans. The explanation may lie in the "always, already, and everywhere social" (AAE) theorem. To be social is to be connected, to evolve connected. We are cognitively coupled by virtue of being socially coupled to others. Compassion and empathy travel across that coupling.

At this point some readers might be wondering about the research on mirror neurons. A mirror neuron fires when an animal acts and when it sees the same behavior in another. Such a mirroring system is supportive of the AAE theorem. The conjecture is that the number of mirror neurons varies directly with the complexity of social life in primates and perhaps in other social animals (e.g., elephants). Brain activity consistent with that of mirror neurons has been found in humans. This is still a very controversial area and I cannot say much more with any confidence. However, some sort of mirror neuron system would seem to be a necessary piece of the social brain puzzle. For a concise discussion of the origins and controversies about mirror neurons, see Rose and Abi-Rached (2013: 140–47; Whitehead, 2008: 122–248).

The first book I came across with the title *The Social Brain* was written by the noted psychologist Michael Gazzaniga and appeared in 1985. Gazzaniga is not the first person to use the term "social brain." To my knowledge, the first use of the term occurred in an unpublished manuscript written by the psychologist B. I. DeVore (n.d.) in the 1950s on the evolution of primates.

The Brain in the Network

Recent developments at the nexus of the social, life, and neurosciences have witnessed the simultaneous invention of network models of systems and subsystems in the brain/mind/culture unit. The first hint of this development for me was the anthropologist Clifford Geertz's argument in 1973 for the synchronic emergence of an expanded forebrain among the primates, complex social organization, and at least among the post-Australopithecine tool-savvy humans, institutional cultural patterns. This statement and his chapter a quarter century later on brain/mind/culture-culture/mind/brain (Geertz, 2000: 203–17) were a significant provocation in my thinking about the brain sociologically in conjunction with Brothers's work.

Another early provocation for my work was Mary Thomas Crane's (2000) *Shakespeare's Brain*. Crane is an English professor who specializes in Renaissance literature and culture. She is representative of the trend toward interdisciplinary scholarship that marks the latter part of the twentieth century. She travels easily over the terrain of her specialty but just as easily in the lands of the cognitive sciences. The thesis she defends in her book is that biology engages culture and produces mind on the material site of the brain. This view articulates the architecture implied in Geertz's view of a network model of brain, mind, and culture.

A new idea like that of the social brain does not appear out of the blue in the mind of one person, in one specific form, or in one location. New ideas tend to emerge as multiples, not singletons. That is, for any given innovation in its early stages there will be themes and variations on the innovation being pursued simultaneously throughout a particular cultural region. Given a certain level of societal need on the one hand and a useful innovation on the other hand, one version will eventually coalesce out of this variety and crystallize as an invention or discovery that enters the society or segments of the society. Sometimes innovations have the potential for wide social applications; sometimes they are narrowly useful for particular occupational or professional communities. So it should be no surprise to find social ideas about the brain bubbling up all over the intellectual landscape initially signalled by Brothers's 1990 paper.

In addition to the people I have already mentioned, consider neuroscientist Leah Krubitzer (2014) and sociologist Bernice Pescosolido (2011). Krubitzer does not offer a specific model but rather a series of lessons learned in her research that have led her to realize that culture has played a key role in shaping our brains and behaviors. She stresses the significance of epigenetic research in redirecting us away from brains in vats to brains in contexts. The network concept shadows every one of the lessons she shares with us.

Pescosolido develops a sophisticated network model of the brain in context. She begins already knowing that the twentieth century ended with many scientists acknowledging the complex entanglements among genes, neurons, and behavior across different time scales. She concludes that we need a framework that links biological foundations, biological embedding, and social embeddedness. She calls that framework the Social Symbiome and develops it on the foundations of a networks and complex systems science approach. The Social Symbiome has a kinship with my social brain model and the connectome. I will discuss and generalize the connectome concept in concluding this chapter.

Pescosolido's model illustrates the multiples hypothesis. In linking the brain to the social environment, she finds herself in the company of philosophers like Alva Nöe (2010) and Andy Clark (1998), the anthropologist Clifford Geertz, the biologist E. O. Wilson (2012), the evolutionary neurobiologist Krubitzer, the evolutionary anthropologist Dunbar (1998), and me, a sociologist/anthropologist. Pescosolido's model is graphically different than mine but links "genes and proteins," "body," "self," "supports," "institutions," and "place" modeled respectively by molecular networked systems, biologically networked systems, individual systems ties, pathways to health/

disease/health care, personal social network systems, organization-based network systems, and geographical systems.

Reigning Myths about the Brain

Let's review some of the persistent myths about the brain that not only impact popular ideas about the brain but continue to guide the research and thinking of many neuroscientists. Due to a misunderstanding and misinterpretation of the earliest split-brain research, it became widely but mistakenly "known" or assumed that we operate within a relatively strict left brain/right brain paradigm.

The left brain is alleged to support mathematical and logical skills; the right brain is supposedly the more artistic side. The brain does in fact have two main segments. They are connected by the corpus callosum, a large bundle of more than two hundred million myelinated nerve fibers and smaller fissures, including the anterior and posterior commissure and the fornix. Hemispheric specialization is not absolute but rather relative and fluid (Roser and Gazzaniga, 2009). The two sides work wholistically, collaboratively, and in a close synchronous dance (Baars and Gage, 2013: 89–108). We think with our entire brain (and, as we will see, with our entire body in its social and environmental contexts). Left brain/right brain thinking is associated with localization theory, the theory that specific sections of the brain control specific functions such as language. Increasingly, neuroscientists have been forced to leave these traditional ideas behind and confront a new reality: culture plays an important role in determining what we do and think, and cognition—or more generally, mentality—does not exist "in" the brain, nor for that matter in the environment, but in a systemic "in-between" space that links brain, mind, culture, and environment. It is important to recognize that this is a conclusion more readily reached if you approach the brain as a social scientist, but it is a conclusion being forced upon neuroscientists by their own research (see Star, 1989, for a sociological study of localization theory in context). Research continues to support localization theory but in increasingly nuanced ways.

Localization in its boldest form claims that different areas of the brain control different aspects of behavior. This concept emerged in the nineteenth century when Paul Broca discovered that damage to the left frontal lobe resulted in speech impairment. In 1874, Carl Wernicke identified "Wernicke's area" in the left temporal lobe as controlling receptive speech. Fritsch and Hitzig had already discovered that different movements of the body could be produced by stimulating different parts of the cerebral cortex. As the neurosciences developed and research tools became more sophisticated, replication of localization studies did not unequivocally support the theory.

Equipotential theory was proposed by critics of localization theory. This theory claimed that all areas of the brain are equally active in cognition. Some researchers (for example, Goldstein and Lashley, cited in Williams and Karim, 2018: 32) argued that basic motor and sensory functions are localized but not higher mental functions.

Let's consider a classical example of brain-centric theorizing about the social brain. This will serve as another instance in this book that helps separate and distinguish what I have achieved from the efforts of others. Graziano (2013) understands the social brain from the inside out. According to Graziano, the brain, "a mere collection of neurons," creates consciousness. The sociological perspective, already evident in Clifford Geertz's writings from the early 1970s, sees consciousness as a social phenomenon arising from the resonances and synchronicities of social life.

Graziano is a neuroscientist, and he uses the tools of his trade to construct an empirically based theory of consciousness he calls "attention schema theory." Understood in its own context, this is a rationally constructed theory by a serious scholar. On the basis of the experimental evidence on social thinking, Graziano draws attention to the two brain regions that repeatedly show up in scans: the superior temporal sulcus (STS) and the temporo-parietal junction (TPJ). Graziano thinks in terms of "machinery in your brain" that participates in social perception. The STS and TPJ are a team that is expert at "attributing awareness to other people" (Graziano, 2013: 11–12, 23): "Awareness is a description of attention." Awareness, Graziano (2013: 37) writes, "is not merely watching, but plays a role in directing brain function." Graziano's (2013: 231) concluding remarks underscore the brain-centric nature of his theory: the attention schema theory "explains how a brain can attribute that particular, complex, rich, idiosyncratic combination of properties to itself, to others, to pets, and even to ghosts and to god."

There were times as I read this book when I thought here is the point where if he'd read G. H. Mead he might see that he was close to a sociological threshold; and there were times as I read this book when I thought here is the point where if he'd read Gilbert Ryle he might see that the brain is not the mind, and that the mind is just the body at work. One of the things we do see in Graziano's theory is certain concepts at work in the postmodern atmosphere of brain studies impacting that theory as they have impacted my theory: complexity, resonance, recursivity, and information. In related literature, we find additional concepts at work, such as network and flow, and changes in the basic forms and substances of the world of humans, fauna, and flora, everything changing from one sort of stuff to another (Gotman, 2012: 77; and see Deleuze and Guattari, 1987).

Rose and Abi-Rached (2013: 233–34) illustrate a widespread imperative to go beyond the illusion of the myth of individualism. At the same time they illustrate how difficult it is to escape the "self-evident" fact that we are ruled by the neurobiology of our brains. They claim on the one hand that we are not "mere puppets of our brains." That's because "we still have mental states, an internal psychological realm of thoughts, intentions, beliefs, and will" (Rose and Abi-Rached 2013: 162–63). So the myth of individualism is still with us! This is not impacted by the "fact" that we all now agree that social factors are important. But how are they important? Are they coupled in co-evolution with the brain or must they "pass through" and "have effects via the brain"? For all their rhetoric on the illusion of individualism, they cannot get past their social neuroscience conviction that all social behavior is implemented biologically. In this sense then having a social brain means having a brain specialized for collective ways of life (Rose and Abi-Rached, 2013: 143). In the end they are prepared to "take seriously the combined assault on human narcissism from historical and genealogical investigations, from cultural anthropology, from critical animal studies, and from neurobiology" to take us beyond the myth of individualism (Rose and Abi-Rached, 2013: 233–34). After all of their schizoid travels between radically social brains and classically biomedical brains, they leave us on the threshold of a very different idea of what a society is, what human freedom is, and what it means to be a human person. I wonder if their failure to make a breakthrough is related to their failure to include sociology in their list of disciplines assaulting our narcissism. What a curious omission for a sociologist. But then we must remember that Rose was originally trained as a biologist and that experience has clearly made him the kind of sociologist who is more firmly driven by the science of biology than by the science of sociology. So while he and his co-author (who has a medical background) take for granted that we humans are social creatures, they are not prepared to go so far as to recognize that we, our genes and neurons, and our brains arrive on the evolutionary stage always, already, and everywhere social. We have social brains, social neurons, and even social genes (see the epilogue to this chapter).

Everyone in the twenty-first century who has struggled with questions of consciousness and the social brain has had to tame the concepts of networks, connections, information, and flows. We have all had to grapple with the complexities at the boundaries that traditionally distinguished brains, bodies, and minds, distinctions that fractured beginning in the latter half of the twentieth century. Relative to my social brain colleagues who have navigated those fractured boundaries in the firm grip of tradition, sociology has helped me to mobilize the fractured boundaries and to create a radically *social* social brain model.

The Chaotic Brain

Chaos is associated in the popular imagination with massive dystopian disorder. But over the last hundred years or so, and especially during the past fifty years, we have learned a new vocabulary across the sciences, the arts, and the humanities. The key terms in this new vocabulary are "non-linear," "fractal," "complexity," "self-organization," "dynamical systems," and "chaos." This new vocabulary emerged as we learned the limits of traditional linear and simple billiard-ball causal models. But the concept of "creative chaos" was already being discussed in the writings of C. H. Cooley (1902), an early American sociologist. He understood it as natural and sporadic. Later theorists conceived it as systematically generated and exploited by encultured human societies (Apter, 1982; Turner, 1982).

One of the key lessons of twentieth-century science and culture was that everything was more complex than we thought. One of the practical lessons of this new understanding is that we now recognize that working in a deliberate heavy-handed way to create order in organizations, environments, and our lives is less useful than drawing on approaches that are more flexible and freewheeling. This lesson has already been incorporated in the tinkering paradigm guiding evolution, as we saw in chapter 3. A short-hand management protocol would recommend a "more is less" approach, focus more on outcomes than on processes, give up the idea of a universal order, and recognize that there is order in disorder and patterns in randomness.

Classically, neuroscientists have sought the causal origins of human behavior at the level of individual neurons (the neuron doctrine), at the level of the neuronal organelle (e.g., the synapse or dendritic spine), or at the level of the neural network. These are micro-level versions of the macro-level idea of the "brain in a vat" and might be thought of as "neuron-in-a-vat" models. In both cases, the brain or its neurons are isolated causal reservoirs that are hypothesized to cause our behaviors, emotions, and thoughts. In general the neuron(s)-in-a-vat model treats behavior in terms of a reflex model—a stimulus-response model. At least since the 1990s it has become apparent that the neuron(s)-in-a-vat stimulus-response model is not up to the task of explaining the complexities of human behavior. Newer approaches have drawn on self-organization theory and non-linear approaches in general, including fractals and chaotic dynamics.

Non-linear dynamics has allowed neuroscientists to identify and study neuronal functioning at the level of the "cooperative neural mass." The implication of this line of research is that cortical functioning is internally self-organized. Perception, for example, is not a passive process in which the brain simply registers whatever stimulates the receptors. Perception begins within the brain in self-organized neural activity that lays the foundation for processing input. Internally generated chaotic dynamics is selective about what receptor activity to accept and process.

In general, then, behavior is interactive; the brain in a sense reaches out toward input and gives it form through a self-organized process of patterning. The brain is the locus for this process which gives form and meaning to inputs. But once again I must stress that this brain work does not take place in isolation from body, culture, and environment. Chaos, once thought to be neurologically pathological, turns out to be essential to the healthy functioning of the brain (Lehmertz et al., 2000; Skarda and Freeman, 1987; Stam, 2005). What once was thought to be "noise" that needed to be filtered and eliminated turns out to be relevant behavioral signaling. Chaotic dynamics operate all across the brain at all levels in a network of functioning systems. They operate as the basal background state that keeps neurons exercised so they don't all die. This makes the stability of the brain independent to some extent of stimuli across the entire brain/body/culture/environment system. Chaos is constitutive of complex networks and essential to the creation and stable circulation of information. In a nutshell, the brain does not just blindly process inputs. It is selective. It can be contrasted with "machines" which use periodic or steady-state dynamics. A chaotic system interacts with environmental input using an internally generated activity pattern. Neuroscientists who have pioneered in and developed this model have taken important steps toward giving us a better understanding of how the brain works. However, things are more complicated even than this. My conjecture is that chaotic dynamics operate in a way that complicates tendencies toward hierarchical organization and promotes heterarchical organization. This applies not just to the brain but to the cell-to-gene-to-neuron and the society/culture/environment system. That system is the unit across which chaotic dynamics operate. And it implies that the human *Umwelt* is not unitary but varies as a function of culture.

The *Umwelt* is the world as it is experienced by specific organisms. Our views through our cultural lenses are as different from each other (at the collective level, not the individual level) as the overarching human *Umwelt* is different from the *Umwelt* of other animals. This enhances the difficulties of cross-cultural communication beyond the centripetal force of compassion and the cultural construction of the "we" and the "they." Our differences are much more profound and resistant to the Other because they are rooted in an *Umwelt*. Umwelts are culturally and environmentally patterned; that is, the differences that matter are the differences between human groups and cultures and between different animal species. Culture is a speciating mechanism; we can speak of cultural species in more or less the same way that we can speak of biological species.

The Anarchic Brain

The idea of a chaotic brain has developed alongside the idea of an "anarchic brain." Anarchy, like the term "chaos," as I use it here, has nothing to do with popular views of bomb throwers, disorder, and the breakdown of the rule of law. Anarchism, as understood in the tradition that stems from Peter Kropotkin, is one of the sociological sciences, and anarchy is a specific form of order, a specific way of organizing lives, organizations, and environments. I first used the phrase "the anarchy of the brain" in 2011 but more as a place-holder for an idea than a substantive idea. I now want to unpack what it means to say that the brain is organized according to the principles of anarchy. It is difficult to discuss the chaotic dynamics of information theory and the brain without some technical details creeping in. We can adopt another perspective that can help explain the meaning and significance of a fine-grained review of chaotic dynamics by looking at the relatively gross level of anarchic organization. The major research based provocation for an anarchic theory of brain activity is the effects of psychedelics, which flatten the functional hierarchy of the brain. This is accomplished by liberating "the influence of information ascending the hierarchy." The result is a brain that can "explore its repertoire of possible states with greater ease" engaging entropic brain activity (Blackburn, 2021; see Carhart-Harris and Friston, 2019, and the critical commentary by Noorani and Day, 2020). There is also fMRI evidence for the anarchic brain (Zapparoli et al., 2015; and see Soresi, 2005).

Students of the brain from inside and outside the neuroscience community have been prompted to introduce the concept of anarchy into their research for a number of reasons. The brain does not have a rigid structure. What I discussed above as chaotic dynamics is reflected in the constant structural modifications observed as the brain responds to internal, environmental, and social stimuli. In my view, this is a stronger and more general basis for the anarchic brain hypothesis than the psychedelic and fMRI studies.

Perhaps the most important development in brain studies in the last fifty years is the recognition that the brain isn't "in a vat"; it is in the world with the body, and it has a world and a body. Philosophers reached this conclusion a little earlier than the neuroscientists, but increasingly we have become aware of the arguments against the BIV model. "I"—meaning the cells environment and society unification diagrammed in my model (Fig. 11.1)—am constantly processing the input I receive from my environment. We adapt to the world through a continuing plastic and analytical activity that characterizes all the systems and subsystems in my model. The plasticity of the brain is reflected in the plasticity of the body but also in the plasticity of all the other elements of the unification. This has to be the case because all systems and subsystems are non-unitarily isomorphic to one another.

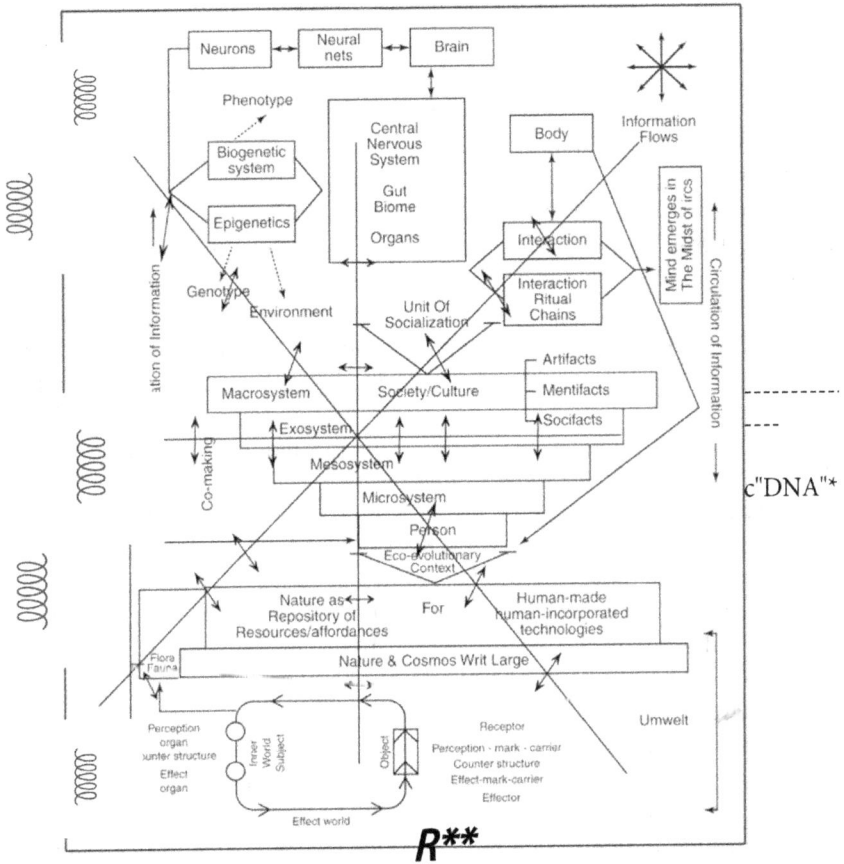

*mechanism for cultural speciation
**universal resonance generator

Figure 11.1. Restivo's Model of the Social Brain.
Source: Created by the author.

Plasticity has its limits in all systems; it inevitably encounters a fundamental recalcitrance in nature. If we analytically distinguish the brain and the body, their adaptability is a function of their plasticity, which at a more fine-grain level reflects chaotic dynamics. The codes underlying the various levels of my model are not rigid. It is this feature of our species that explains our individual and collective abilities to adapt to the world, elaborate it, imagine it, and in a sense create it. However, the codes are constrained by natural parameters that represent the recalcitrance of the world. The mistake some scientists and others make is to assume that the lack of rigidity and the operation of chaotic dynamics is a basis for thought and action without limits.

We can say this in another way. Complex systems operate in accordance with precise rules, but they are so numerous and varied that they cannot be captured in a few laws or equations. Hidden in the search for a Theory of Everything or a single Equation of the Universe is the search for a God-surrogate. This is a lost cause.

What we have in reality is a general uncertainty principle reflected in brain studies and in my model. It might be possible in principle to copy and reproduce the chemistry and structure of the brain, but it would be impossible to copy and reproduce the electromagnetic content, the information circuits, of the brain. We cannot hope to fill in all and perhaps any of the data (information packets, information quanta) that represent our living thoughts and feelings. These are distributed throughout my model; they are not located entirely in the brain. Chaotic dynamics and being in and having a world define a self—a social self to recall my earlier remarks—that cannot be cloned from DNA or discovered in the tissues of a dead brain.

We are talking about open systems that are not deterministic but, as parts of a recalcitrant cosmos, always lawful. The genetic code organizes a framework within the brain and the body in the world, and that framework gets its shape and content from living beings acting in that world. The locus of our "living thoughts and behaviors" is not the brain per se or the body per se; the locus is the brain/mind/body/culture system operating in the world, in an environment of interactions with others and the physical and natural world. If we could have started here, it would have been obvious why Einstein is not only not his brain, he is not even "Einstein." Einstein is only Einstein as a living being acting in the world through a defined period of time and space and moving in and through social networks. One could consider this as another example of Becker's concept that there is no such thing as "the work itself" (see chapter 7). All we have are the many occasions in which behaviors, thoughts, and emotions are performed. We can also consider applying Becker's Principle of the Fundamental Indeterminacy of the Work. The sociology here is the study of how brains and bodies in the world are made and remade. The creative act of making bodies and brains in the world is a labor process and a collective one at that.

If for analytical purposes we once again isolate the brain as a system with agency, we notice that one of its key characteristics is the search for patterns. Once it recognizes a pattern it creates a kind of "information bowl" into which it throws any input that matches, more or less, that pattern. Input that doesn't match is either blocked or subjected to Procrustean forces to make it match. Chaotic dynamics keeps shaking up the bowls so patterns reign but do not rule despotically. This is crucial to creative thought. One of the most important behavioral causes and reflections of chaotic dynamics is humor. We can imagine it working in the following way. Humor shakes up tendencies toward rigidifying patterns of thinking and behavior. It tosses the information in a brain bowl into a mixer. The result is at least a temporary novelty in our experience that is "recorded" as the contents of the bowl as they return more or less to their original configuration. In a sufficiently creative situation of self and context: that configuration never in fact returns fully to any original configuration. It is interesting now to consider all of this in relation to my discussion of improvisation in chapter 7.

There is a playfulness that many of the great scientists recognize to be a piece of doing science. Einstein certainly had this quality. The Nobel physicist Richard Feynman (1999: 199) put it this way: if you're going to work hard on a problem, you have to convince yourself that the answer is "over there." This predisposes you to a certain path. In order to stay the course but allow new information to reach you and possibly alter your path, you have to be laughing in the back of your mind at what you're doing.

Toward a Model of the Social Brain

My model is designed to graphically represent and expand Geertz's remarks on culture and the brain: the expanded primate forebrain, complex social organization, and institutional cultural patterns among the post-Australopithecines emerged and evolved more or less synchronously. This idea anticipates recent arguments for the coupled evolution of brain, mind, environment, and society.

This perspective recommends against treating biological, social, and cultural parameters as serially related in a causal nexus. Rather, these levels should be viewed as reciprocally intertwined and conjointly causal. The claim in a nutshell is that human behavioral repertoires emerge from the complex parallel and recursive interactions of molecules, cells, genes, neurons, neural nets, organs, biomes, the brain's various regions, the central nervous system, other elements of the body's systems and subsystems, and our social interactions in their ecological and *Umwelt* contexts. This implies that we need to rethink socialization.

Socialization is traditionally understood to operate on the person. My model reimagines socialization as a process that simultaneously informs and variably integrates the biological self, the neurological self, and the social self to construct personality and character. In addition, each element in the model must be understood as a dialectical entity containing its own internal "seeds" of change and as following a temporal dynamic that may be at different times synchronous or dyssynchronous relative to other elements.

Each element is conceived as an information system, with all systems multiply interlinked by the circulation of information. All systems, subsystems, and elements of the model are implicated in every thought and action but to different degrees and strengths at different times. They all have causal potential. In the case of a particular failure, a departure from the norm, a deviation in thought or action, the dominant mechanism(s) in explaining the failure, departure, or deviation is only a subset of the system or a particular configuration of elements. The entire network is technically involved, but the peripheral causalities can—again, to different degrees in different cases—be essentially ignored. They are in general "incidental" in the sense that the causal connection to the dominant locus is the one to focus on. The correct subnetwork is the one that isolates the central relationships that allow us to understand what has causal priority. Among all the things going on, where should we intervene if we want to fix what's wrong? If something goes wrong with your car, you don't anticipate rebuilding and reconfiguring the entire car.

Some recent findings on how the brain is structured will eventually have to be taken into account as my model evolves in relationship to research across the sciences. In trying to understand the complexity of the brain some scientists have tried to associate it with something they are familiar with. Scientists at Aberdeen University mapped the brain network to the universe. This allowed them to identify high-dimensional objects that are the key to understanding structure and function. They used algebraic topology to model these structures in a virtual computer-generated brain. The results were then tested on real brain tissue (Dean 2018; Markram, 2008; Reimann et al., 2017). They found that the brain reacts to a stimulus by building then razing a tower of multidimensional blocks on various geometrical scales from rods to planks to cubes (that is from one to three dimensions and on to higher dimensions). This progression is analogous to building a multidimensional sand castle (the "castle" is better described as "materializing") that then self-destructs. One of the structural implications of this viewpoint is the localization of memories in higher-dimensional cavities.

In a related exercise, Vazza and Feletti (2020: 1) compare "the network of neurons in the human brain" to "the cosmic web of galaxies." In other words, the "distribution of matter in the universe looks a little like the *connectome*, the network of nerve connections in the human brain" (Hossenfelder, 2022: 170). The analysis by Vazza and Feletti (2020: 8) is part of a search for "more powerful and discriminating algorithms to pinpoint analogies and differences of these fascinating systems, almost at the conceivable extremes of spatial scales in the universe." Hossenfelder warns against concluding from this study that the universe is a giant brain and thinks, an idea incompatible with the laws of physics. I discuss the nature and applications of the connectome idea later in this chapter.

The dotted diagonals in my model represent a global basal chaotic function based on my earlier discussion of chaos and the brain. The cDNA symbolizes the social brain's relationship to the process of cultural speciation. The *R* represents the universal resonance generator that is the source of the energy for the rhythmicity associated with all the elements of the model. And the coil symbols along the borders represent the sending and receiving mechanisms that generate the field that carries emotions and consciousness in the moments of the mutual co-presence of humans. The model was developed against the background of the research and theory on the social brain. This is a graphic representation of a new way of thinking about the brain in the world and in culture and society.

The Social Brain Model

I have taken this model through several revisions in order to keep current with the most recent developments in the relevant sciences. The model was initially based on an argument for the social brain proposed by the anthropologist Clifford Geertz. He argued, as we have already seen, that the following features of life emerged together, in synch with each other: (1) expanded forebrain among the primates, (2) complex social organizations, and (3) at least among the post-Australopithecine tool-savvy humans, institutional cultural patterns. This perspective implies that we should not treat biological, social, and cultural factors as serially related; that is, we should not think in terms of biological factors causing social factors which in turn cause cultural factors. Instead, the implication is that these factors matter, but they are complexly interrelated in terms of causation. They should be viewed as reciprocally intertwined and conjointly causal. The claim in a nutshell is that human behavior emerges from the complex interactions of genes, neurons, neural nets, organs, biomes, the brain and central nervous system, other elements of the body's systems and subsystems down to the molecular level (see Pert, 1997), and our social interactions in their ecological contexts.

The unit model is activated in a triad of unit models and it is that triad that is the basic model of brain/mind/culture/world. This reflects the idea that the triad, not the dyad, is the basic unit of social life.

Connectomes

The latter part of the twentieth century can be described as the age of the network, an era in which thinking began to be dominated by the idea of connections. In 2005, Olaf Sporns and Patric Hagmann, exemplifying the principle of multiples, independently introduced the term "connectome" to refer to a map of the neural connections within the brain. They were inspired by the effort to construct a genome, to sequence the human genetic code. More generally a connectome maps the elements and interconnections in a network. Connectomes may range in scale from maps of parts of the nervous system to the neural connections in the brain. They have been used specifically in connection with mapping the neural connections in the brain. Partial connec-tomes have been constructed of the retina and primary visual cortex of the mouse. In line with these developments, my model represents a connectome of connectomes. The next stage in this project is to construct the triad unit of my model, three interconnected individual models, and then to embed this triadic connectome in the nested networks of the social and cultural connec-tomes locally, regionally, and globally. I visualize a global connectome driven by the circulation of information across a global network of nested networks. This sounds complicated, but we're talking about a complex network model of the peoples, flora, fauna, and ecological systems and subsystems of our planet. On the rationale for a global connectome (my interpretation), see Khanna (2016). Some progress has been made recently on using connec-tomics to predict behaviors.

The first wiring diagram of a pinhead-sized (one-cubic-millimeter) piece of human brain tissue was recently completed. It produced 1.4 petabytes worth of images (Shapson-Coe et al., 2021). The first full-brain wiring diagram was completed more than thirty years ago for the roundworm (White et al., 1986). The roundworm has only 302 neurons in its brain. The process took fifteen years to complete. It is now possible to diagram a roundworm brain in about a month. In a recent study, the connectomes of eight genetically identical roundworms from larval to adult were constructed. As much as 40 percent of their connectomes differed.

Connectomics is becoming a critical resource in neuroscience. In prin-ciple, connectomes are a key, in terms of the reigning neuro-paradigms, to understanding how the organism thinks, feels, moves, remembers, perceives, and so on. So far, however, it hasn't been much help in explaining how the brain functions. That would involve at least parsing the overwhelming inter-connectivities in the complex brains of humans and non-human primates. Connectomes also tell us nothing about the quality of the connections they map. They indicate a connection between neurons but not whether the con-nection is strong or weak. For this and other reasons involving, for example, the activity of neuromodulators, we should not expect connectomes alone to explain brain functions.

I take note of a recent study in human brain connectomics based on graph-based mathematics that found striking interhemispheric asymmetry and intraparcel heterogeneities (Hanalioglu et al., 2021). The authors are careful to note that their findings might be the result of artifact or technical errors. They are more persuaded that their use of data science and optimi-zation applications are key methodological contributions to future studies in network neuroscience. If these findings turn out to be robust, they will offer some evidence of localization but of the type defended by Goldstein and Lashley (as discussed earlier) on split-brain functions. In any case, we shouldn't expect to find universal patterns of localized or hemispheric functions. Rather, we should expect any evidence of localization to reflect specific network patterns of the systemic movements of bodies through time, space, culture, and the environment.

Consider now a conceptual formula for the probability of an "innovative thought." This will look more technical than it really is. My objective in constructing this formula is to try to isolate the factors that go into predicting creativity, or more realistically the probability of a creative thought. The formula for the probability of an innovative thought (iTp), then, should look something like this: $iTp = qc^2 (K+G)$, where qc^2 is the amount of cultural capital the person commands and K is a constant that represents the cultural context and network structure the person is embedded in; qc^2 because doubling the amount of cultural capital, for example, quadruples its impact factor. $K = C + Nt$ where C = Cultural Context is an index that takes into account a variety of demographic and institutional diversity indicators; N = the density and diversity of the network structure of the society at time (t). G = the genius cluster quotient at time (t). When considering the etiology of behaviors that are traditionally considered genetically grounded, it is now important to recognize that the brain, like humans, arrives on the evolutionary stage always, already, and everywhere social. Therefore, what we have considered to be linearly transmitted genetic phenomena must now be viewed in the context of a brain that is at no stage of development separated from the social and cultural imperatives that form us. The very notions of "genes" and "genetic" must now be revised in the context of the social brain model. Genes and neurons are social entities.

Some recent studies that do not rely on social brain or connectome models demonstrate that there is a rationale for pursuing the advanced network directions of the work I've been drawing your attention to. They demonstrate two things: one is that there are indeed information flows that link the brain to the organs of the body; the other is that the links between the brain and the liver, heart, and gut are notably stronger than other links. One researcher argues that the heart, for example, thinks for itself; rather than waiting for instructions from the brain, it sends signals to the rest of the body on its own. In fact, the heart sends more signals to the brain than the brain sends to the heart.

The gut-brain axis has long been recognized as a key linkage. Gut bacteria make 90 percent of the brain's neurotransmitter serotonin and a variety of neuroactive compounds. The brain sends signals to the gut that stimulate or suppress digestion. The brain's connection with the liver is notably complicated (Bruce et al., 2017; Gao et al. 2017; O'Hare and Zsombok, 2016). The lesson of such studies is that the most complicated object known to humanity, the brain, does not do its work alone. And the connections, as I've indicated, reach outside the body into the world around us, including our social relationships. Researchers in neuroscience have been exploring the vagus nerve, which forms a complex network linking the brain and the internal organs. This network is being viewed as shaping thoughts, memories, and feelings. This network is implied in my model (Underwood, 2021).

Is Plato the Second Coming?

I am obliged to pay attention to recent developments in brain-machine inter-action and brain-computer interaction (BMI and BCI). This work, exem-plified by Miguel Nicolelis's (2011) research and development program, involves experiments with the wireless transmission of thoughts. It promises life-changing cognitive prosthetics. At the same time I see a troubling resur-rection of an ancient Platonic dream (or nightmare) of "free-floating minds," minds freed of the flesh. Nicolelis imagines minds without bodies, or with bodies that do not have to move, communicating "wirelessly" across a room, a city, a country, a continent, the galaxy. The ancient fear of the flesh we see here is at bottom a fear of the female flesh. This is a sign that science is still being fueled by patriarchy and the masculine fear of the feminine.

If all of the research and theory I have been rehearsing in this book points to a social self, a social mind, and a social brain, where is "the social" in BMI and BCI? Decades of work in science and technology studies have dem-onstrated that the social and more broadly the cultural are embodied in the hardware and algorithms that make the machines in this work function. But wireless transmission seems to violate the basic principles of social construc-tion. There is a technology at work here—wi-fi technology—and not ESP. Sociologist and STS scholar Jennifer Croissant of the University of Arizona (and my former PhD student) argues (personal communication) that these wireless results will only work if and to the extent that the participants have a set of shared kinesthetic and cultural references (e.g., relative homogeneity in brain mapping and information processing, starting with the linguistic level). Just as we can no longer assume transparency in everyday communications as diversity in all its varieties increases, so therefore these systems will either be extremely narrow in their potential participants and applications *or* have to engage a model of the social brain and an enormous amount of cultural complexity in algorithmic form so that there is interoperability amongst diverse brains. As diversity increases, the amount of effort spent indexing communications increases. More and more metadata and contextual data will be needed to understand if two interlocutors are talking and thinking about the same thing.

Cultural diversity will pose huge challenges to complex BMI and BCI, but even the relatively narrower diversity characteristic of individual brains will overload bandwidth and algorithms. At the same time, my introduction of a field feature of social selves and social brains opens up new avenues for "wireless" communication in face-to-face and face-to-interface configurations.

From Elixirs of Life to Digitized Minds:
The Flawed Logic of the Quest for Immortality

Digitized minds, BIVs and simulations share a basic theme. That is the extent to which they are part of the most recent efforts by humans to achieve immortality. We should know by now that this is a mad scheme given the fact that immortality is not part of the future of the Cosmos as we understand cosmology today. But nonetheless, a search for the elixir of life was already an objective of the first emperor of China, Emperor Qin (third century BCE), Emperor Wu (Han Dynasty 206 BCE–220 CE), and later Taoist alchemists during the Six Dynasties period (third to sixth centuries CE). The latter developed an elixir containing toxic substances such as mercury sulphide and arsenic sulphide. The lower classes were unable to take such dangerous paths and turned to medicinal wines and diets. Modern Chinese continue to be influenced by the myth of Chang'e, the goddess of the moon, associated with an elixir of life over two thousand years ago. Her name appears on a popular brand of dietary supplements (Kong, 2022). Chinese mythology also references the Peaches of Immortality, thought to be the elixir of life of the immortals.

Western alchemy sought after the philosopher's stone, a substance that could turn base metals into gold or silver. It was also known as the elixir of life, capable of giving eternal life. The Fountain of Youth, a mythical restorative spring, was already found in the writings of Herodotus (fifth century BCE). Chemical sources of elixirs of life were superseded during the twentieth century by biological elixirs. Cloning and cryonics became "scientific" as opposed to alchemical paths to immortality. As technology surged into the digital age, the technogods began to speak of "digital immortality" and created a "digital afterlife" industry. On the broadest scale of the immortality scenario, we in the West have gone from the biblically inspired notion of conditional immortality in an afterlife dependent on salvation to a technoscience promise of salvation on Earth (Hentsch, 2004). Rosenberg (2022) offers several technological objections to the very possibility of a digitized afterlife.

Looking at this through the lens of the social self/socal brain-in-the-world, the quest for immortality fails the test of reason on so many levels that it appears to be a mad dream and nothing more. You couldn't clone a new Einstein from his DNA without taking the next step and replicating every instance of Einstein's real life. Nor for the same reasons could you digitally clone an Einstein who would live forever while the original Einstein passed away.

CONCLUSION

The research frontiers in the neurosciences are moving very rapidly and brain researchers are regularly announcing new and surprising discoveries. As a neuroscience watcher, I'm alert to the fact that developments even within the BIV neuroist framework could radically alter our understanding of the social brain. It's hard to say in what ways or directions, but there are still so many things we don't know about the brain per se that it is not unreasonable to expect changes that will impact my model coming from newly discovered features of the brain. I am confident that however radical these changes are they will not overturn the basic message of my model and social brain thinking: our interactions and environment impact the brain. Stay tuned.

EPILOGUE: SOCIAL BRAINS, SOCIAL GENES, AND HUMAN ONTOGENY IN CULTURAL EVOLUTION

The social brain is an innovation. It should be expected that in a culture so attuned to the neurosciences as our own that efforts will sooner or later be made to produce popular introductions to the social brain. This has already happened in the case of self-help books based on the biological brain. We are now seeing books on the market that are aimed at introducing the social brain idea to the public and to "sell" the ways in which this innovation can be useful to individuals and organizations. My book is different from all the other social brain books and blogs on the market by virtue of its grounding in sociology.

The competing titles are written primarily by psychologists who are oriented to social neuroscience. Social neuroscience is an interdisciplinary field devoted to understanding how biological systems implement social processes and behavior, and to using biological concepts and methods to inform and refine theories of social processes and behavior. Thus, the focus in that literature is on the priority of biological systems over and against social systems. The competing literature take for granted the "emerging" idea that we are radically social creatures. I put "emerging" in quotes because our radically social nature has been known to sociologists for almost two hundred years. Contemporary social brain authors give priority to biology, psychology, and neuroscience and pay little or no attention to sociology. Therefore, their concept of the social is not as powerful as the strong sociological approach I advocate. To elaborate, consider the difference between psychologist Michael Gazzaniga's concept of the social brain and anthropologist Clifford Geertz's concept of the co-evolution of the brain and culture.

Gazzaniga (1985) made the bold move of linking biological and cultural forces in a serial causal nexus. He argued that causal forces determining our behavior and thought arise at the biological level and progress through the social and cultural levels. That viewpoint has prevailed into our own time among those neuroscientists who have actually taken social and cultural factors into account in their theories. When he comes around to explaining a specific complex human behavior, religious behavior, Gazzaniga falls back on a biological theory that is not informed by social theory. This is typical of the way psychologists approach the social brain. Social brain biologists also give priority to the biological over the social. The biologist E. O. Wilson (2013) doesn't specifically refer to the social brain, but he makes the best argument by any scientist, including sociologists, for the radically and uniquely social nature of human beings. But, like Gazzaniga, when he turns to explaining a complex social institution like religion he falls back on a biological explanation.

The contrast with Geertz's (1973) argument for the synchronic emergence of brain, society, and culture and his theory of brain/mind/culture-culture/mind/brain (Geertz, 2000) is clear. Geertz is the primary stimulus for the network model of the brain in culture and environment I developed with Sabrina Weiss in the 1990s. The social brain psychologists and neuroscientists favor nexus models that linearly link biological and social causes. It's important to understand the way in which my approach is radically different from that of the social brain biologists, psychologists, and neuroscientists. There's certainly some overlap, including in the way we think about practical everyday applications. I discuss these overlaps in the next chapter.

The idea that our genes are social is suggested by the research on the "cooperative gene" (which should be contrasted with Dawkins's concept of the "selfish gene"; Attwater and Holliger, 2012; Ridley, 2008; Roughgarden, 2009; Vaidya et al., 2012). This research is independent of the "always, already, and everywhere social" concept I argue for. This would synchronize the cooperative gene with the cooperative principle that operates on all levels of life and all levels of the organism. Gottlieb's (2007: 1) concept of "developmental manifolds" may be relevant here and to the rationale for my social brain model; the probabilistic epigenesis framework "emphasizes the reciprocity of influences within and between levels of an organism's developmental manifold (genetic activity, neural activity, behavior, and the physical, social, and cultural influences of the external environment) and the ubiquity of gene-environment interaction in the realization of all phenotypes." In *The Selfish Gene*, Dawkins (1976) defends the classical gene-centric theory of evolution: the more two individuals are genetically related, the more sense (at the level of the genes) it makes for them to behave cooperatively with each other. The book is considered one of the most influential science books of all time, according to a poll taken in conjunction with the thirtieth-anniversary celebration of the British Royal Society's science book prize (Armistead, 2017). Dawkins (2006) appeared to take a step back from this gene-centric position when he wrote in the foreword to the thirtieth-anniversary edition of the book that he should have titled his book "The Immortal Gene." But in fact he was comfortable with his original thesis, only emphasizing that the book was more about altruism than selfishness. If he had given altruism a sociological transformation, he might have hit on the concept of the cooperative gene. I am grateful to David Moore of Pitzer College for sharing his views on this matter in a personal communication (see Moore, 2001).

Human ontogeny occurs uniquely by comparison to other animals "in a culturally-evolved world. . . . The culturally constructed environments of human ontogeny likely affect how we think and perceive the world in fairly deep ways. This means that our 'cognitive architecture' will evolve non-genetically through our interaction between culturally-evolving environments and our ontogenetic learning processes that allow, at least in part, our brain's cognitive architecture to adapt to the circumstances of the current generation. This also implies that people who experience different cultures will have different brains" (Henrich, 2008: 24). Furthermore, this leads me to consider that the same principles apply to within-culture differences based on class, ethnicity, sex, and gender.

NOTE

1. The literature on the social brain in theory and practice encompasses a large and diverse literature. In some cases, classical brains-in-a-vat and neuroist assumptions find their way into new social brain theories. Clark (1997) is a philosopher. He does not deal with the social or sociology (these terms do not appear in his index). It's possible that he imagines the social is enfolded in his treatment of "environment" (something he suggested to me in a conversation over coffee), but this is not the same as taking social life and sociology into account explicitly. Noë (2009) is a philosopher and he understands that the brain is "in the world." He addresses social ideas (socially distributed cognition, social presence, and sociolinguistic environment) but seems totally ignorant of sociology as the science of society and proposes *biology* as the science of society. Hayes (2018) is a psychologist who travels something like a progression from "the brain" to behavior. After the first few chapters the approach tends to be more integrative but stays the psychological course. Swart, Chisholm, and Brown (2015) combine expertise in applied neuroscience, psychiatry, and organizational psychology. They want to shed light on the interactions of brain, behaviors, beliefs, and attitudes. The focus is on brain chemistry and individual behavior. The foundational sciences for the authors' systems approach to leadership are cognitive science and physiology. Siegel and Bryson (2012) assume the brain "pretty much determines who

we are and what we do." The book is about the "whole-brain child" and the "child's developing mind." Like many writers on the brain, journalists and brain scientists alike, the authors don't always distinguish between "mind" and "brain." Richard Lopez's blog (2010), *Our Social Brains*, is an example of the neuroscience perspective on the social brain. This blog also exemplifies the prominence of psychologists as proponents of the neuroscience perspective. The blog's headline is *Our Social Brains—Why the neuroscience of social phenomena matters*. Lopez has the same objective that I do: to demonstrate why social brain research matters to us in our daily lives. Notice that Lopez asks why the neuroscience of social phenomena matters, as opposed to my approach: why the sociology of social phenomena is what really matters. Perhaps the book that comes closest to mine in terms of objectives and audiences is Lieberman (2013). We agree that we need to do more to protect and enhance the conditions that reinforce our social nature. That social nature can be undermined, for example, by creating conditions that make us focus on material goods and money instead of relationships, to cultivate and crave material security at the expense of friendships. In brief then we both stress that we are more social than we know, we have social brains, and this has practical implications for our daily lives. He does not understand the concept of humans as always, already, and everywhere social, and he does not argue for the radical inseparability of brain, mind, body, self, society, culture, and environment. We are at one in offering readers substantive alternatives to the majority of brain self-help books which do not put as much stress as we do on the social brain and the social self. Lieberman's discussion of the need for friends is weakened because he doesn't understand friendships as interaction rituals. Our approaches are as different as sociology and psychology, and sociology and biology. Nonetheless, it is possible that our books could be complementary. Cozolino (2012) is on the right track in terms of bringing psychotherapists up to date on the latest neuroscience, but he doesn't deal with the science of social interactions. Bartra (2014) is an important scholarly contribution but dedicated to saving free will. He is naïve from a sociological and neuroscientific perspectives. Graziano (2013) understands the social brain from the inside out. According to Graziano, the brain is nothing more than a collection of neurons and that is the source of consciousness. The sociological perspective, by contrast and already evident in Clifford Geertz's writings from the early 1970s, sees consciousness as a social phenomenon arising from the resonances and synchronicities of social life. Decety (2020) adopts a developmental perspective on the social brain with a focus on the biology of social cognition. Hood (2012) understands the self as a product of our relationships and interactions but argues that the self exists only in our brains. In his view we are our brains. Slaby and Gallagher (2014) exemplify the concept of "socially extended minds." Their "critical neuroscience" says that the mind does not reside entirely in the brain or the body. Clark and Chalmers (1998) stress the active role of the environment in driving cognitive processes. As I noted earlier Clark is not insensitive to the level of social analysis and theory I bring to the study of the brain, but he buries whatever he understands about the social in the concept of environment. This won't do. But these authors are clearly on the right track. The human subject is not an isolated biological entity. It is coupled to other biological individuals as well as various "cognition-enabling institutions, tools, procedures, and practices" (Slaby and Gallagher, 2014: 21). These authors caution neuroscientists not to mistake the individual biological system for the full human person. The full scope of the human mind must encompass cognitive-enabling institutions, mind extensions, and social-normative practices. The extended mind concept does not fully embrace a sociological understanding of the brain as a social and cultural entity, but it is an important step in going beyond neuroism and the myth of individualism.

Chapter 12

The Social Brain in Health and Illness[1]

We are the most radically social of the social animals. We have social brains. Now what? The social brain concept is already changing the way we think about the brain in health and illness. There is a growing literature on how the social brain concept affects our views of autism, Alzheimer's disease, and how we practice clinical psychiatry (Restivo et al., 2020). The social brain also challenges the brain self-help industry, which has produced many books, exercises, and pills that are supposed to enhance brain function. This industry is based on the idea of the brain as an independent biomedical organ. The social brain model suggests that we can enhance our mental lives and the health of our brains by focusing on our social lives. Keep in mind that I am not distinguishing individual actions from social actions. The key distinction when thinking about the social brain is between loneliness and togetherness. Alone time is not the same as loneliness. For example, there are benefits to meditating with others as well as meditating alone. There are specific kinds of recommendations like this based on sociological principles that can positively influence brain health given the social brain paradigm. Since the social brain does not eliminate the biomedical brain, medical interventions are still relevant. However, medical interventions will have to begin to acknowledge the social brain.

This chapter addresses the increasing awareness that "bowling alone" and "loneliness" are literally killing us and provoking violent behavior. Understanding our radically social selves and our social brains can help reverse these trends. Current regimens and protocols for enhancing cognition are based on the traditional biomedical model of the brain and are thus highly problematic. It is important to gain some perspective on these enhancement regimens now that we understand that we have social brains.

We saw in chapter 2 how biomedical assumptions about the isolated brain drove important initiatives in the United States (Bush 1990 and Obama

141

2013). Similar initiatives were undertaken in the European Union, Japan, Saudi Arabia, China, and elsewhere. I also drew attention to one of the few counterpoints to these programs, the Brains in Dialogue workshops I participated in held at various European venues between 2009 and 2011. These dialogues were strongly interdisciplinary and even included sociologists and neurological patients. The public has not been educated to follow and support such interdisciplinary efforts. Instead, they have been directed to think along traditional lines by the colorful images created by neurotechnologies such as fMRIs (functional magnetic resonance imaging) and PET (positron emission tomography) scans. These images "show" the brain in action doing things like playing chess, reading words, and even helping to locate God in the brain (the God spot) and the place in the brain where our morals reside. In the midst of all this have come calls for new models, theories, and agendas in neuroscience and mental health services, including psychiatry. How does all of this affect you in your everyday life?

One thing to keep in mind before we move on is that the relationship between brain images and behavior is not at all firmly established. Dumit's (2004) study of the nature and cultural ramifications of PET scans and Joyce's (2008) study of fMRIs in the landscape of consumer medicine imaging were early warning signs from the science studies community about these technologies. A recent report in *Nature* (Callaway, 2022) reports that "studies linking features in brain imaging to traits such as cognitive ability could be too small to be reliable." The study referenced is Marek et al. (2022; and see Mackenzie, 2022, on the replication crisis in neuroscience).

It's important to consider alternative ways of treating the brain in health and illness, and different and more realistic everyday pathways to self-improvement and enhanced brain functions. Before we go any further, it's important to recall our earlier discussion about the fact that selves, minds, and brains are not defined in "one-size-fits-all" terms. The fact that individuals are social does not erase their cultured and biological individualities. Selves, minds, bodies, and brains are sexed, gendered, raced, classed, and otherwise reflections of the stratifications that define a society. The social inequalities and social injustices that come with social stratification can also impact biology, and humans are subject to biological accidents at and after birth. As we discuss principles of caring for "the social brain," let's keep in mind that putting them in practice will involve adjusting "doses" to the needs and backgrounds of particular individuals. This is becoming more common in general medicine as a goal if not always in practice yet. For example, research has been underway since the early 2000s on tailoring drug dosages to individual genetic profiles (e.g., Goldstein et al., 2003; Haga and Burke, 2004; Ware, 2012; and see the literature on neurodiversity: Doyle, 2020).

The public relations of the brain in society are being carried out in a BIV context. That is, the public has been sold a view of the brain as an independent biological organ that controls all of our behaviors, thoughts, and emotions. It is from this perspective an organ subject exclusively to medical interventions. From the 1990s to the present, this view of the brain has fueled a self-help industry promoting brain-enhancing pills, behaviors, exercises, and technologies. How useful are these enhancements? Let's keep in mind that snake oils are as American as apple pie. They gain credibility in the context of the myth of individualism, America's anti-intellectualist history, the pathologies of advertising, and pathological views of what it means to be "free."

CAN PILLS ENHANCE YOUR BRAIN FUNCTIONS?

The social brain paradigm does not erase the biological brain or medical interventions. The social brain incorporates the biological brain into its network. The biochemical system of the social brain can be and is altered by chemical inputs from everyday foods to exotic drugs. So, drugs in the form of pills or liquids can in principle affect the social brain. What do we know about brain-enhancement drugs? The medical conclusion is that there is not enough evidence to support spending money for brain-boosting supplements. Americans spend close to one hundred million dollars a month on such supplements. One of the most popular supplements is ginkgo biloba. A study published in the preeminent medical journal *Lancet Neurology* looked at three thousand adults seventy years and older who were complaining about memory functions. The study found that gingko biloba did no better than a placebo in reducing rates of developing Alzheimer's disease. In similar studies DHEA (the hormone dehydroepiandrosterone) supplements also proved to be ineffective. Neuriva, a pill marketed for its alleged brain-enhancement properties, is being pitched in TV ads by an actress who happens to have a doctorate in neuroscience but is not a practicing neuroscience researcher. The Neuriva company has withdrawn its early claims about the supplement's scientific and clinical foundations. The actress spokesperson has stopped claiming that Neuriva is part of her brain health routine. This is all part of an out-of-court settlement in the case of Neuriva's manufacturer versus several plaintiffs. Gary L. Wenk (2020), a professor of psychology and neuroscience at Ohio State University, referred to Neuriva as snake oil. In March of 2022, an eight-million-dollar false-ad class-action agreement between Reckitt Benckiser LLC and Neuriva consumers won final approval after a federal judge in Florida adopted a magistrate's earlier recommendation. Consumer advocates suggest you'd do better, based on better science, eating berries.

Other top-selling brain enhancers include LumUltra, Brain Pill, Alpha Brain, and Prevagen. The science behind these products and their effectiveness in practice are still under review. The FDA *has* approved Aduhelm (aducanumab) for the treatment of Alzheimer's using the federal agency's accelerated approval pathway, which can be used for a drug that provides a meaningful therapeutic advantage over existing treatments for a serious or life-threatening illness. We are still a long way from establishing the long-term effectiveness of these treatments, and for the moment they should be approached with reasonable caution and skepticism and always with the advice of personal physicians.

It's important to emphasize that the social brain paradigm does not invalidate the biochemical structures and functions of the brain, so some drugs could in principle enhance brain functions. B vitamins have performed well relative to placebos in reducing cognitive decline. Supplements of these natural ingredients, in particular B-12, are only necessary if your doctor determines your levels are low. You need to proceed with caution here since high doses of B-6, for example, can reduce kidney function and lead to strokes. Curcumin, which is found in the spice turmeric, has been shown in some studies to benefit thinking and memory. Again, caution is advised since many commercial brands have less of this compound than indicated on labels. Other supplements that have shown signs of improving cognitive functions are cacao flavanols, found in chocolate (caution is needed because many cocoa powders are contaminated with cadmium, a heavy metal), and fish oil, which is a widely used supplement. Eating fatty fish such as tuna, mackerel, or salmon a couple of times a week should supply all the fish oil you need. Supplements have not shown the same cognitive effects as including fish in your diet. Vitamin E was advertised and used as a supplement for decades. It was promoted for increased energy and sexual performance. It also showed some cognitive benefits in some studies. Recent research has raised questions about its effectiveness and safety, and it certainly doesn't show any evidence of preventing or reducing the symptoms of cognitive decline. Finally, a recent study "shocked" researchers by showing evidence of the cognitive benefits of multivitamins. The authors cautioned that they are not ready to conclusively concretize and generalize their findings (Baker et al., 2022).

The effectiveness of brain-boosting supplements is controversial at best, and the overall results of independent and commercial research should not instill confidence in consumers. In principle, supplements can be effective for cognitive enhancement. But you shouldn't use them without consulting your personal physician or neurologist. And if you know how to use online sources and the library critically, you should do the research needed to help make informed decisions about whether particular supplements are right for you in consultation with your physician.

One final piece of information on this topic. According to Harvard Medical School's online *Harvard Men's Health Watch* newsletter, brain-booster supplements, like other over-the-counter supplements, are not regulated by the US government. There is no solid proof any of these supplements actually work. There are some suggestions for improving cognitive function and avoiding or mitigating cognitive decline that apply equally to traditional models of the brain as well as to the social brain model. These include aerobic exercise and a plant-based diet.

Aside from supplements, diet, and exercise what are some of the general suggestions neuroscientists have for maintaining brain function? Harvard Health Publishing lists several ways you can help maintain healthy brain function and reduce the risks of cognitive decline. *Mental activities* create and strengthen connections between nerve cells and can even lead to the generation of new cells. Reading, taking courses, doing puzzles, and tackling math problems are examples of activities that stimulate your brain. These activities take advantage of our newfound understanding of neuroplasticity: the brain has a built-in capacity for change. Physical activities like drawing and painting and craft activities also contribute to brain health. This takes advantage of body/brain integration. *Physical exercise* increases the number of tiny blood vessels that bring oxygen-rich blood to the brain, especially to those areas of the brain traditional research assigns to thought. New cells are developed, and connections across brain cells increase. All of this takes advantage of the innate plasticity of the brain, resulting in greater efficiency and improved adaptivity. The general impact of exercise on overall health—lower blood pressure, cholesterol levels, and blood sugar balance—also contribute to brain health. Maintaining good blood pressure and controlling high blood pressure are key factors in cognitive health. Controlling blood sugar can help you avoid diabetes, an important risk factor for dementia. The same holds for high levels of LDL cholesterol. *Good eating habits* are of course a key part of mental and physical health regimens. Many recommendations for diets that support brain health mention the Mediterranean diet, which emphasizes fruits, vegetables, fish, nuts, olive oil (unsaturated), and plant-based proteins, and the DASH diet, rich in vegetables, fruits, and whole grains. It includes fat-free or low-fat dairy products, fish, poultry, beans, and nuts. It limits foods that are high in saturated fat, such as fatty meats and full-fat dairy products. In the past, some physicians recommended a *low-dose aspirin regimen* to reduce the risk of dementia, especially vascular dementia (this refers to reducing the blood supply to the brain). This idea has come under scrutiny recently. The chances of bleeding in the stomach, intestines, and brain on an aspirin regimen are now considered too high, especially for persons over 60. *Avoidance regimens* include, notably, all types of tobacco and alcohol. Some studies indicate that there can be health benefits to drinking alcohol in moderation;

this means, for example, no more than two glasses of wine a day. Some studies suggest any level of alcohol intake is detrimental to your health. You are advised to avoid anxiety, depression, sleep deprivation, and exhaustion, which are important health goals in general even though they do not clearly predict the risk of cognitive decline.

Interestingly, the last item on the Harvard list is "build social networks." This would be the first item on my list. The social brain model aside, strong social ties are associated with lower risk of dementia, lower blood pressure, and longer life expectancy. As the first item on my list, it modifies all the other items by recommending that wherever possible, heathy activities should involve others at least some of the time.

Enhanced Environments

One of the first signs of a new approach to brain health that eventually linked up more strongly with the social brain model than the traditional biological brain model was observations about enriched environments. Yuan et al. (2012; and see Li, et al., 2021), for example, demonstrated that an enriched environment improved cognitive abilities in mice. The idea that stimulating environments enhance cognitive performance can be traced to research in the late 1940s that found rats raised as pets were better problem solvers than rats raised in cages. In the early 1960s, single rats in cages were compared to groups of rats in cages equipped with toys, running wheels, ladders, etc. Researchers first discovered that the rats raised in the enhanced environments showed increases in a certain enzyme activity. It was soon learned that these environments increased the volume of the cerebral cortex. This increase was later found to be the result of increased thickness of the cerebral cortex and greater numbers of synapses and glial cells. The classical studies by the Harlows in the early 1960s on maternal and social deprivation in rhesus monkeys demonstrated the significance of social stimulation for normal cognitive, emotional, and sexual development.

In recent years, scientists have been able to link the enhancement effect to changes in the three-dimensional organization of chromosomes in the neurons and glial cells of mice brains. The genes related to human brain health are notably impacted by these changes. From the perspective of the social brain model, it is important to note that the enhanced mice were raised in groups exposed to stimulating environments. The controls were raised in smaller groups in unenhanced environments. Genomic comparisons with humans show that the three-dimensional changes in mice brains parallel regions of the human brain associated with complex cognitive traits such as insomnia, schizophrenia, and Alzheimer's.

Part of the conspiracy of mythologies that define contemporary ideas about brains and selves is the assumption that the neurosciences hold the keys to solving all of our mental, behavioral, and emotional health problems, and perhaps our social problems as well. In chapter 2, I introduced this approach as the "neurological fix."

Putting the Social into the Social Brain

We have now established a strong rationale for considering how our social environment impacts the structure and function of our brains. This is not a rationale for ignoring biochemical and electrical interventions. It is a rationale for exploring ways in which social variables under our control in our everyday lives can be used to enhance our cognitive functions and protect and heal our own brains. As we begin to think about ways to reimagine our social lives in the context of the idea that we are social bodies with social selves carrying social brains, certain existing and novel strategies come into greater focus.

We hear a great deal about meditation in the context of keeping the brain healthy (Horowitz, 2010). Meditation has been shown to strengthen the prefrontal cortex. This is important from a classical perspective because localization theory in neuroscience tells us that this is the area of the brain we use in decision-making and planning. Localization theory has been going out of fashion in recent decades, and certainly the social brain paradigm implies a more holistic distribution of brain functions. A holistic distribution doesn't negate the possibility that certain brain regions may carry more of the burden of a behavior, emotion, or thinking process. In any case, it seems clear that meditation is brain-health positive. Its effectiveness is increased if we practice meditation with others some of the time. Instead of or in addition to sitting meditation, Thich Nhat Hanh and Nguyen Anh-Huong (2006) recommend walking meditation. By incorporating walking meditation into a daily or weekly schedule, every step can be part of a deeper practice of interbeing. This is a spiritual interpretation which can be adapted to secular practices.

Walking meditation is a physical activity you can practice alone and with others anywhere indoors or outdoors where there is enough space to take a few steps. There are four basic stages in doing walking meditation: (1) Pick a safe, distraction-free space in which you can move comfortably. (2) Take ten to twenty steps in a straight line in a deliberate, slow, rhythmic way, turn around, and repeat. (3) Pay attention to the movement of your legs and how they feel as you lift and lower them. Be mindful of any other feelings you are experiencing. It is normal for your attention to begin to wander. You can bring back your focus by listening to your steps and your breathing. There may be noises in the area that you can't block out. Acknowledge them and refocus on your breathing, your steps, and the movement of your legs. (4) As with any activity, including sitting meditation, practice is required and you can make faster progress if you make ten to fifteen minutes of meditation walking part of your everyday routine. Having a partner will enhance the benefits of the activity.

Here is a summary of what we know to various levels of certainty about everyday products and practices that have been shown to enhance cognitive functions: (1) The caffeine, L-theanine, and catechins in *green tea* may enhance cognition and act as a dementia preventive. (2) The anthocyanins in *berries* can have a positive protective impact on the brain. (3) The nutrients in leafy greens such as vitamin E (controversial), flavonoids, and folate have been linked to better brain health. (4) A regular *sleep routine* can reduce toxins that promote Alzheimer's. (5) Your brain needs input. Make *learning new things* a routine part of your life. This provides fuel for basal brain activity and cell activity in general. It strengthens connections across neurons and fuels neurogenesis. (6) Some studies have shown that *yoga* increases the volumes of the frontal cortex and the hippocampus. By decreasing stress, yoga contributes to reducing the risk of memory loss and dementia. (7) Hydrate. Chronic dehydration is a factor in cognitive decline. (8) We all know by now that *exercise* is an important factor in promoting healthy aging and longevity. What many people are not sufficiently aware of is that exercise is only beneficial if you practice "rest and recovery." The same is true for brain work, thinking. Thinking is only beneficial if you practice mental "rest and recovery."

You've had ample opportunity as you've read through this book to realize the importance of a rich *social network* even if it's a network of two people (for example, a couple, married or not, related or not, same sex or not) who live together. Studies have shown a relationship between more social interactions and slower rates of memory decline and lower rates of age-related cognitive decline. If you live alone, a rich virtual network (connections with people you rarely see because they live too far away) and an active creative life can help, to some extent, to make up for the lack of a strong face-to-face network. If you are so inclined, volunteering, joining clubs, and participating in sports and cultural activities have been shown to improve overall health. Screen time is not a substitute for face-to-face interactions.

Understanding Social Connections

Let's begin with some basic definitions. *Social isolation* is the relative absence of social relationships. *Social integration* refers to the overall level of involvement in social relationships. *Formal social relationships* take place in organizational environments (e.g., religious institutions, volunteer settings, business environments). *Informal social relationships* take place in the home and neighborhood (having a spouse, friends, and acquaintances). Earlier I discussed this in terms of secondary (formal) and primary (informal) relationships. The *quality of relationships* can vary from positive (emotional and other forms of support) to negative (conflict and stress). *Social network* refers to the web of social relationships. Social networks can be stronger or weaker and vary by density, sheer numbers, and other variables. I will review in the next section the ways in which the quantity and quality of social relationships affect physical and mental health and mortality risks (Umberson and Montez, 2010).

Mortality rates are greater for individuals with the lowest level of involvement in social relationships. This is true even when we take socioeconomic status, health behaviors, and other variables into account. Social relationships also lower mortality risk among adults with health issues such as coronary artery disease. More generally, the degree of involvement in social relationships has been shown to impact the risk of preclinical conditions. Studies have shown that low levels of social interaction and relationships are linked to cardiovascular disease, hypertension, cancer, delayed recovery from illness, recurrent myocardial infarction, atherosclerosis, autonomic dysregulation, inflammatory biomarkers, and impaired immune functions. Marriage is the most studied social relationship. Studies show that marital history shapes various health outcomes, from cardiovascular disease to chronic conditions and depression.

Why do social ties matter? The answer rests ultimately on one of the basic themes of this book: humans are always, already, and everywhere social. There is no controversy about the positive relationship between social ties and general health. This relationship exists because social ties or networks influence behaviors that impact our health. Being married (with some caveats) tends to promote good health because spouses are able to monitor and facilitate their partner's health. Religious ties work the same way, not because of belief in God or an afterlife, and not because there actually is a God and an afterlife, but because religion is a community and family affair. All such networks work to our benefit because they serve as pathways to information and norms that can and do influence our health habits.

Research across various disciplines and populations demonstrates that mechanisms like social support and symbolic meanings promote health. The connections that link these mechanisms are more important than any single mechanism. With respect to specific mechanisms: (1) Social support: being loved, cared for, and listened to benefit physical and mental health. (2) Symbolic meaning: group identity can influence behaviors that may be good or bad for our health; meanings attached to the institution of marriage and families, peer groups, racial and ethnic identity, socioeconomic status, sex, and gender impact how we understand and mobilize health norms. They also impact institutional availability and access to health information and health care. (3) Mental health and physical health reinforce each other even in traditional brain/body models; social ties can enhance emotional ties and have a positive impact on mental and physical health.

Traditional biomedical models of the relationship between society and health have already set the stage for the more pronounced understanding of social ties and health in brain/body/culture/world models. Because social ties are so central to our mental and physical health and well-being, stresses and strains in those ties can be very damaging to our mental and physical conditions. Extended periods of stress, conflict, and depression will cause cumulative wear and tear on those biochemical and electrical systems that contribute to our health and well-being. The impacts of stress, conflict, and depression show age-related differences. For example, stress in young adults is associated with alcohol consumption and with weight gain in mid-life adults. Social contagion is a factor in one-on-one and group relationships. A risk-taking spouse can cause the other spouse to consume more alcohol. Obesity in a spouse or a friend can lead the other spouse/friend toward obesity. Poor social ties are also associated with poor compliance in regard to medical regimens and protocols.

In a society with smaller families, an aging population, and poor safety nets care for the elderly increasingly involves family members. This can be doubly problematic. Caregivers may become stressed and this may negatively impact them and the recipients of that care. Caring for elderly spouses or parents is associated with poorer health in both the provider and the recipient. Social ties are a constant of our lives. There may be some optimum level of social ties relative to our health and well-being, and perhaps too many social ties may not be beneficial. In any case, it is abundantly clear that the fewer those ties the worse for our health and well-being. The effects of social ties are constant in the sense that they are always impacting us. But they can vary in immediacy, intensity, and cumulative impact over a lifetime.

In a classic study of suicide, Emile Durkheim (1897/1952) sought to explain what appeared to be a random individual behavior, suicide, in societal terms. By studying suicide rates, he was able to demonstrate a causal connection between community solidarity and individual suicides. Egoistic suicide was the result of not being integrated in a community. The individual suicide is prompted by the feeling of not being tethered to a well-defined source of meaning and support. Altruistic suicide, by contrast, is caused by an excessively high level of integration into a group. Suicide in such situations would follow from group norms, values, and beliefs of the sort we find in cults and in military service. Anomic suicide follows from moral confusion and lack of direction, notably during times of societal upheavals. A rapid rise in stock market prices is as likely to provoke suicides as a rapid decline in prices. Fatalistic suicide is the opposite of anomic suicide. Durkheim considered this a theoretical category without real-world occurrences. But a prisoner who was subject to constant abuse and excessive regulation might be a candidate for fatalistic suicide. Durkheim concluded that suicide rates are higher in (1) men than in women (with the exception of women who remained childless for years); (2) those who are single as opposed to those in an intimate relationship; (3) parents without children versus parents with children; (4) Protestants, followed by Catholics and then Jews; (5) soldiers as opposed to civilians; (6) peacetime than during times of war; and (7) Scandinavian countries by comparison with other countries. In general, the defining context in each of these cases is the degree of social solidarity.

There are a variety of reasons to criticize the research behind these findings. Some critics believe Durkheim committed the ecological fallacy. This is a formal fallacy in the interpretation of statistical data that occurs when inferences about the nature of individuals are deduced from inferences about the group to which those individuals belong. He was also criticized for his methods of drawing and using data. After we sort through all of the criticisms and controversies we are left with a legitimate insight: strong social integration, social ties that are not overwhelming, is in general not conducive to suicide. We can look back from this perspective on our discussion of loneliness, ill health, and violence.

The cumulative advantages and disadvantages that characterize social groups across race, class, ethnic, gender, sex, and power differences are societal factors that impact our individual and collective health and well-being. So are inequalities in social ties. Very little is known about variations in social ties across sociodemographic groups, but sociologically we should expect variations. We do know about certain differences that are associated with race, gender, social class, and education. These are outside of our individual control and require the attention of policy makers and funding agencies at all levels of government and the private sector. All other things being equal, the more informed and up to date policy makers, politicians, civic leaders, and funding agents are the better able they will be to address the societal variables that affect our individual and collective health. Bringing their neuroscience knowledge up to date in terms of the social brain should be a top priority of science advisors and knowledge influentials. This is a huge problem because it involves revealing and repairing the myth of individualism which is built into the fabric of American culture. This would also require bringing sociology into the corridors of power and policy in a more direct and visible manner than now seems possible. Bringing social-tie perspectives and findings into the policy arena may lead to more cost-effective ways of improving individual and collective actions to address issues of the brain in health and illness. Because of the ways in which social networks function, we can expect multiplier effects to follow on social-tie policy initiatives. This can have a large impact on prevention as well as reducing our dependence on drugs and technological interventions which are expensive and come with side-effects. There will be side-effects as we widen the scope of our social ties interventions, but they are likely to prove less lethal and more readily reversed than those associated with drugs and technologies.

Policy Perspectives

We have enough scientific support today for recommending policy initiatives that can foster improvements in preventive and curative protocols in a brain understood as a social and cultural system. I want to focus on the contributions sociological thinking about the brain can make to these policy initiatives. These turn on what we know about the brain health benefits of social ties, connections, and networks. We know that social relationships play a role in brain health and illness and affect mortality risk (Umberson and Montez, 2010). They can be a foundation for promoting brain health and general health across entire populations. Social relationships should be recognized as a public health resource and should be supported by specific offices and departments in public and private funding, policy, and oversight agencies. There should be a priority investment in individual, collective, and public health.

Social relationships have a dark side, and this should be recognized in constructing policy initiatives. Relationships can become strained, conflictful, abusive, and alienating, and their positive and negative aspects are unequally distributed across socioeconomic and sociodemographic groups. Since these stresses are impacted by social inequalities and social injustices, correcting those inequalities and injustices becomes an imperative in public health policy.

Policies that reflect the provocations of the social brain paradigm and more generally the realization of the dangers of social isolation are already coming online. Health and Human Services, a government agency in America, has introduced a "marriage initiative" based on the principle that positive marriages facilitate health and well-being. We can bracket the ideological motivations here and recognize this as a "relationship initiative." Such policies should embrace marriages and sustained relationships among lesbian, gay, bisexual, transgender, questioning, queer, intersex, pansexual, two-spirit (2S), androgynous, and asexual individuals. Attention should be given to the fact that one-size-fits-all programs are likely to help some people and harm others. The poor and elderly are at greater risk for social isolation than other populations, and this should be reflected at the policy level. Hospital and insurance policies that promote or otherwise force people into home-based medical care place more of a burden on women, minorities, and those with diminished social and economic resources.

The dangers of social isolation have increasingly come into focus. The COVID-19 pandemic has underscored the research findings on this topic. Addressing social isolation and the classic problem of alienation means putting our educational and community resources to work in ways that provide safe public spaces for group activities and compassionate attention to those who have been isolated due to the loss of family members and other loved ones (for example, the widowed). The principle "do no harm," often attributed to the ancient Greek Hippocrates (of the Hippocratic Oath) but more likely a nineteenth-century construction, should become a community norm across all our institutions. It should apply in work and school environments as well as medical ones. This should be part of an effort to coordinate social-tie strategies across the helping services. This is not an argument for "safe places" for ideas or for eliminating offense in education.

These are all matters of great urgency given demographic trends that include smaller families, high divorce rates, homeless populations, an aging population, and various employment-related issues. All of these factors foster social isolation.

CONCLUSION

All of the behavioral and policy protocols I've discussed in this chapter cannot be tackled using conventional medical models. They require a transformative approach to our mental and physical problems at the societal level. We are not talking about a new medicine, an innovative surgical technique, a new diet or exercise program. What is required is a new understanding of what it means to be a society, a community, a family, a worldwide community of communities. We must figure out a way to remake our society, our culture, our global village on the foundations of the principle that we humans are always, already, and everywhere social. We must understand compassion, empathy, and belongingness as societal prescriptions for health and well-being. All of this is complicated beyond our capacity to imagine by the existential threats we face today as a species and as a planet. There is a reason our media, new mythologies, and storytelling are dominated by dystopian images. We appear to be collectively overwhelmed by the reality of the threats we face. More than ever in our history we are aware of the fragility of our place in the cosmos. It's one thing to learn to cope with death and dying, to imagine the ultimate extinction of our species and of our planet thousands to billions of years from now. It's quite another to face the immediacy of climate change, the death of ecological niches, the pollution of our air and water, and the disappearance of bees and frogs. Terrible scenarios seem more imminent than hopeful ones. But at least we have better ideas about what to do and what not to do. These are still embedded in individuals and relatively small segments of our populations. Until and unless they reach the hearts and minds of the most powerful agents in our political systems or become championed by mass movements on a scale we have not yet seen in human history, we will continue to slide down into a worldwide arena of disasters. It's time to start turning off some of the lights, literally and figuratively.

NOTE

1. The views I express on medical and non-medical protocols and regimens in this chapter are based on independent research which draws in part on the following source materials: GCBH (2019); Grand View Research (2022); Harvard Health Publishing (2022); Onaolapo, Obelawo, and Onaolapo (2019); and Ricci (2020). The term "nootropics" was introduced by Giurgea (1972). Giurgea and Salama (1977) expressed some optimism about the future application of these drugs as brain enhancers. This optimism showed up in other studies during the latter part of the last century. More recently, the most positive conclusions suggest caution. Concerns have also been expressed about ecotoxicity issues arising from the increasing popularity of these drugs (e.g., Wilms et al., 2019).

Chapter 13

Final Considerations

BRAIN, SOCIETY, AND SOCIOLOGY

I have indicated at various points in this book that we are in the midst of an era of multiplicities, pluralities, complexities, and transformations in categories and classifications that have reigned for millennia. I have argued against one-size-fits-all conceptions of brain, mind, and self. Perhaps I have not made this clear enough. I am predisposed to general theory and to the values associated with Marx's vision of communism, White's (1977: 173) Merlin the magician's advance beyond communism to anarchism, Nietzsche's concept of the "Overman" understood as self-actualization, and Kropotkin's stress on mutual aid and anarchism. These roots branch out widely and wildly into interdisciplinary and postmodern postcolonial feminist networks. I have reflected on the varieties of sexual orientations, my opposition to patriarchy and masculinism, and the need to attend to the variety of ways in which race, ethnicity, class, sex, gender, and culture impact the relations between societies and brains and the structural outcomes of those relations. Moreover, as a sociologist of science I'm aware of the ways in which "objective" science is vulnerable to the prevailing values of the society it is embedded in.

This is just part of the picture. The inner organizational cultures of the sciences also condition their objectivity. I first drew attention to the sociology of objectivity in a 1974 paper (Restivo, 2022: Chapter 5). Nonetheless, in drawing on the findings of the various sciences that bear on my study of the social brain it is easy to forget this or at least to forget to alert the reader to what the issues are. Pitts-Taylor (2016) has drawn attention to ways in which neuroscience ideas about plasticity and mirror neurons, for example, are conditioned by neoliberal hype. This doesn't automatically obviate the scientific materialism and realism of these concepts. But it's a good reminder that scientific facts of the matter come with a caveat emptor warning, which I alerted you to in my prologue.

OPEN SYSTEMS THINKING AND
SCIENCE REDUX: A REVIEW

No particular study, concept, lab result, scientist, or scientist's claim is scientific by itself. The science is teased out over generations. In this respect, I have no trouble identifying myself as a scientist, a materialist, and a critical realist. I do not see any evidence for free will and precious little for agency. The appearance of agency is a function of the fact that we are complex open systems. All systems are more or less open. There are no absolutely closed systems anywhere. However, to the extent that any given system is closed, to that extent the system will allow for predictions. In that sense all systems are as deterministic as they are closed. All systems, however, are lawful (Bohm, 1957).

Universals and invariants are distributed across the varieties of bodies, brains, selves, and cultures. Social constructionism is not, as so many uncritical observers contend, the claim that scientific objects are "theorizable only in representational terms as the effects of discourse" (Pitts-Taylor, 2016: 19). As the fundamental theorem of sociology, it states in materialist and realist terms that humans have only one way to discover and invent, and that is by way of their social interactions with others in social contexts embedded in earthly ecologies. This applies to all human beings, abled, disabled, classed, raced, sexed, gendered, and cultured. In the same way, the principles of mimesis and entrainment apply to all human beings. This means that we need to be, as Pitts-Taylor is, sensitive to the fact that brains, bodies, and selves (and the sciences that study them) are situated in social, biological, and ecological inequalities. All humans are members of a species that is always, already, and everywhere social. Culture can and does intervene, enhance, fracture, and fragment evolutionary realities and introduce and/or strengthen conflict, inequalities, and violence, factors that interrupt social and emotional energies and communications. Nature itself is not free of these factors. Pitts-Taylor (2016) is right to warn us about the tendency in neuroscience to hype the science around positive and constructive interventions. We saw in chapter 7 that this is also the case in robotics where the emphasis is on constructing sociable, cuddly, friendly robots and not social robots who could become Virginia Woolf or Nietzsche, who could become cognitively or physically disabled, who could be classed, raced, sexed, and gendered.

What do communism, anarchism, the Overman, and mutual aid mean in this context? The general values, norms, beliefs, and action they entail must contend with inherent differences that make a difference in the human condition. We can either give up at this point and step away from those realities that make change for the better utopian or mad, that allow differences to obstruct invariance where it rules, or we can press on with the understanding that our projects for improvement must engage the pluralities, multiplicities, and varieties of brains, bodies, selves, societies, and cultures. This has implications for our age of identity politics.

The "I" is a grammatical illusion. We are multitudes. We are living in an age of flux in categories and classifications. And yet we see movements to essentialize our identities. We find ourselves fixing our sexual and gender identities, resisting challenges to those identities, seeking fixed selves that require liking and respect. These movements have sacrificed becoming to being. But what is "becoming" in a world without free will? Nietzsche urged us to overcome our selves, to resist the external forces that label us and the internal forces that enslave us to those external forces. He was not as sharp as Marx in recognizing our socially constructed selves, but he understood that we are shaped by history and environment. Without free will, without anything as powerful as Nietzsche's Will to Power, how do we avoid essentializing labels?

The fact is that we can't escape labeling. Culture is a labeling activity, a way of establishing and sustaining order. For the self to be in flux, for our identities to avoid fixation, we need to live in societies that are complex, evolving, generating more and different social networks for us to travel through. If there are societal and geographical limits to this process, we need to press on through the arts and our imagination. We need to be and to cultivate open systems at every level, from bodies and selves to societies and ecosystems. Our adaptability depends on that. We don't achieve this by way of free will or the Will to Power but by collectively tinkering through, not so much using past experience and the fund of knowledge, but flowing through them. We are dependent on many factors over which we have no control, but we can know things and we can act accordingly, not freely, but out of necessity. Culture by way of language is inherently essentializing. Every word essentializes. This is especially true to the extent that our languages are noun based. A more "becoming" language might be constructed on the foundation of verbs (as suggested by Bohm, 1976). Some Native American languages are verb based in the sense that they contain a lot of verbal morphology for verbs but very little for nouns. Root forms are typically verbs, and noun forms are often expressed by adapting a verb or using a phrase. Unlike English, in which abstractions are typically expressed as nouns, Cree, for example, has "Tell the truth" as a simple verb. This might give some weight to Bohm's propositions taking cultural context into account. It is easy in these circumstances to be drawn into a spiral of disturbing contradictions. Is there a way out?

What we think and do are consequences of our movements through social, cultural, and environmental spaces and times. Pay attention to the way thoughts "come to you" unbidden. We don't think but rather become aware of thoughts generated by the interactions between our apparatuses of consciousness and the affordances of our environs. The sense of self and of self-awareness emerges at the nexus of the streams of consciousness and the streams of affordances. I have borrowed and adapted the concept of affordances from a decidedly complicated literature on the subject. Gibson (1966) introduced the term and defined it as "action possibilities in the environment." Norman (1988) introduced the concept into the human computer interaction literature and defined it as "perceived properties that may or not actually exist." Gaver (1991, 1996) separated affordances from their perceptive qualities in an effort to clarify the various ambiguities of the concept (see the reviews in Soegaard, 2015, and Kaptelinin, 2014). Thoughts, to construct a slogan, are after-thoughts.

I have to admit to an internal struggle that arises as I write these words between my sense of free will and my knowledge of the fallacy of introspective transparency. Can we resolve this with greater clarity about thinking, doing, and willing?

Classically as in our own time it has been widely assumed in lay, scientific, and especially philosophical circles that we humans consciously, systematically, and rationally will our own thoughts and actions. Langer, Blank, and Chanowitz (1978) are among many who have questioned that assumption. Neuroscience research from the 1960s to the 1990s, capped by Libet's (e.g., 1985) controversial research on "unconscious cerebral initiative," provided the provocation behind recent headlines claiming that neuroscience proves free will is an illusion. The neuroscience in this arena remains controversial.

Philosophers like Daniel Dennett (2014) and Alfred Mele (2014, 2017) have pointed out the many different definitions of free will, and Dennett believes that at least some common conceptions of free will are compatible with neuroscience findings. We have also witnessed the emergence of a research literature on "automaticity" (Bargh and Chartrand, 1999: 462). The three major forms of automaticity are: (1) "an automatic effect of perception or action," (2) "automatic goal pursuit," and (3) "a continual automatic evaluation of one's experience." These various unwilled systems perform the lion's share of the self-regulatory burden, grounding the individual in his or her environmental currents. These ideas go against a history of two-stage models of free will that have been proposed by writers from Willian James to Karl Popper and Daniel Dennett to Roger Penrose. The psychologist Donald T. Campbell's "blind variation and selective retention" concept is an example of a two-stage model of free will: first chance, then choice; first "free," then "will." Thoughts come to us freely; actions go from us willfully. Hu, Park, and Roskies (2021) offer a new interpretation of the neuroscience data that undermines its challenge to free will. These two-stage models are designed to save free will, but they reflect the fallacy of introspective transparency, ignorance of automaticity, and a failure to account for or even acknowledge social and cultural programming.

In the interest of addressing social problems of inequality and injustice, well-meaning activists and policy makers have morphed those problems in ways that essentialize body, self, sex, and gender, and created "safe place" ideologies that have transformed public forums and universities into places that threaten intellectual freedom. In my own teaching career, I was criticized by some students and some administrators for questioning the taken-for-granted, sanctified authority of religious beliefs, political beliefs, economic beliefs, sexual beliefs, and beliefs about free will, values, and morals. This violates the idea that everything is and must be in motion and the priority of becoming over being (*cf.* Bohm, 1957). At the end of the day, we are obliged to act "as if" we have free will when we find ourselves "choosing" even though we understand that this is an illusion. The university classroom should protect the bodily safety of students; it should not be a safe place for ideas, values, and beliefs. Salman Rushdie warned us that without the freedom to offend there can be no freedom of expression (Martino, 2022). And Nietzsche (1878/1996: Chapter 9, para. 483: 179) remarked that "convictions are more dangerous enemies of truth than lies."

CONCLUSION

I have done my best to provide a first approximation to a model of the social brain that has the power to guide us in a positive direction without making it a fool's errand. I am not convinced that this is possible. We are living as I write this in a world where the faults in our biology; our brains, bodies, selves, and cultures; and our local, regional, and planetary ecologies are strained to a point that has us on the verge of a series of earth-shaking events that threaten to destroy our species and our planet.

In the best and the worst of times everything is in flux. Every word and concept in this book is in flux. Every scientifically established fact of the matter is in flux. We've already seen that knowledge claims escape their evidence, and how we can still know things. A recent headline announced (not for the first time): "Objective Reality May Not Exist at All, Quantum Physicists Say." But don't let your guard down. You should still look both ways when you cross the street in New York, read the directions below the curb when you cross the street in London, and be prepared to look six ways when crossing the boulevards of Rome and Paris.

Two things: First, objectivity is not a monolith; it is shaped by culture, and different groups live in different objectivity communities. Second, principle of the profundity of the surface, but remember that this is a portal to the objectivities of "other worlds" like the worlds of quantum physics and relativity theory, not to mention the worlds of certain judges and political leaders. Look both ways when you cross the street, my friends. That is a "definitive prescription."

What could I be missing? Could there be a myth of the social or a myth of the cultural that stands side by side with the myth of individualism? Is there an Einsteinian revolution waiting to transform sociology, anthropology, and social psychology? I cannot embrace this possibility, but I am not so foolhardy as to claim there is nothing new waiting for us around the next social science turn. Such a possibility would no more overturn Durkheim than Einstein overturned Newton. The "social" would no more disappear than "gravity" disappeared. Remembering that the theory of relativity is a theory of invariance, we cannot rule out a "social and cultural relativity" revolution. Stay tuned.

Bibliography

Aldous, J. (1972). "An Exchange Between Durkheim and Tönnies on the Nature of Social Relations with an Introduction by Joan Aldous." *American Journal of Sociology* 77, no. 6: 1191–200.

Alger, H. Jr. (1868/2017). *Ragged Dick: or, Street Life in New York with the Bootblacks*. Midland Park, NJ: Pinnacle Press.

Apter, M. (1982). *The Experience of Motivation: The Theory of Psychological Reversal*. New York: Academic Press.

Aral, S., and M. Van Alstyne (2011). "The Diversity-Bandwidth Trade-Off." *American Journal of Sociology* 117, no. 1: 90–171.

Armistead, C. (2017). "Dawkins Sees off Darwin in Vote for the Most Influential Science Book." *The Guardian*, July 20.

Aspers, P. (2007). "Nietzsche's Sociology." *Sociological Forum* 22, no. 4: 474–99.

Attwater, J., and P. Holliger (2012). "The Cooperative Gene." *Nature* 491: 48–49.

Baars, B. J., and N. M. Gage (2013). *Fundamentals of Cognitive Neuroscience*. London: Academic Press.

Baker, L., et al. (2022). "Effects of Cocoa Extract and a Multivitamin on Cognitive Function: A Randomized Clinical Trial." *Alzheimer's & Dementia*, July 10: 1–12.

Bandyopadhyay, A. (2019). "Resonance Chains and New Models of the Neuron." Available at: https://medium.com/@aramis720/resonance-chains-and -new-models-of-the-neuron-7dd82a5a7c3a.

Bardy, C., et al. (2015). "Neuronal Medium That Supports Basic Synaptic Functions and Activity of human Neurons in Vitro." *Proceedings of the National Academy of Sciences* 112, no. 20: E2725–34.

Bargh, J. A., and T. L. Chartrand (1999). "The Unbearable Automaticity of Being." *American Psychologist* 54, no. 7: 462–79.

Barlow, A. (2013). *The Cult of Individualism: A History of an Enduring American Myth*. Santa Barbara, CA: Praeger.

Baron-Cohen, S. (1995). *Mindblindness: An Essay on Autism and Theory of Mind*. Cambridge, MA: Bradford.

Barr, J. (2000). "Biblical Criticism." In *History and Ideology in the Old Testament: Biblical Studies at the End of a Millennium*, pp. 32–58. New York: Oxford University Press.

Barton, J. (2010). *The Bible: The Basics*. New York: Routledge.

Bartra, R. (2014). *Anthropology of the Brain: Consciousness, Culture and Free Will*. Cambridge: Cambridge University Press.

Bassetti, C., and E. Bottazzi, eds. (2015). "Rhythm in Social Interaction." *Etnografia e Qualitativa* 8, no. 3.

Bauchspies, W., J. Croissant, and S. Restivo (2006). *Science, Technology, and Society: A Sociological Approach*. New York: Blackwell.

Beaulieu, A. (2000). "The Brain at the End of the Rainbow: The Promises of Brain Scans in the Research Field and in the Media." In J. Marchessault and K. Sawachuck, eds., *Wild Science: Reading Feminism, Medicine and the Media*, pp. 39–54. London: Routledge.

Beaulieu, A. (2001). "Voxels in the Brain: Neuroscience, Informatics and Changing Notions of Objectivity." *Social Studies of Science* 31, no. 5: 635–80.

Beaulieu, A. (2003). "Brains, Maps and the New Territory of Psychology." *Theory and Psychology* 13, no. 4: 561–68.

Becker, H. S. (1982). *Art Worlds*. Berkeley: University of California Press.

Becker, H. S. (2006). "The Work Itself." In Becker et al., eds., *Art from Start to Finish*, pp. 21–30. Chicago, IL: University of Chicago Press.

Becker, H. S., R. A. Faulkner, and B. Kirshenblatt-Bimblett, eds. (2006). *Art from Start to Finish*. Chicago, IL: University of Chicago Press.

Bell, J. S. (2012). "The Performativity of a Historical Brain Event: Revisiting 1517 Strassberg." In M. M. Littlefield and J. M. Johnson, eds., *The Neuroscience Turn: Transdisciplinarity in the Age of the Brain*, pp. 49–70. Ann Arbor: University of Michigan Press.

Benn, D. J. (1972). "Self-Perception Theory." In L. Berkowitz, ed., *Advances in Experimental Social Psychology*, pp. 1–62. New York: Academic Press.

Beretta, M., M. Conforti, and P. Mazzarello, eds. (2016). *Savant Relics: Brains and Remains of Scientists*. Sagamore Beach, MA: Science History Publications.

Berger, P. (1963). *Invitation to Sociology*. New York: Anchor Books.

Berger, P., and T. Luckmann (1966/1991). *The Social Construction of Reality*. New York: Anchor Books.

Berliner, P. F. (1994). *Thinking Jazz: The Infinite Art of Improvisation*. Chicago, IL: University of Chicago Press.

Bettelheim, B. (1986). *Surviving the Holocaust*. New York: HarperCollins Flamingo.

Bivins, J. C. (2015). *Spirits Rejoice! Jazz and American Religion*. Oxford: Oxford University Press.

Blackburn, G. (2021). "LSD and the Anarchic Brain." *Psychedelic Science Review*, June 10. https://psychedelicreview.com/lsd-and-the-anarchic-brain/.

Block, N. (1998). "On a Confusion about a Function of Consciousness." In N. Block, O. Flanagan, and G. Guzeldere, eds., *The Nature of Consciousness: Philosophical Debates*, pp. 375–415. Cambridge, MA: MIT Press.

Bloor, D. (1987). "The Living Foundations of Mathematics." Revision of Livingston (1986), "The Ethnomethodological Foundations of Mathematics," *Social Studies of Science* 17: 337–58.

Bohm, D. (1957). *Causality and Chance in Modern Physics*. Philadelphia: University of Pennsylvania Press.

Bohm, D. (1976). *Fragmentation and Wholeness: An Inquiry into the Functins of Language and Thought*. New York: Humanities Press.

Bostrom, N. (2003). "Are You Living in a Computer Simulation?" *Philosophical Quarterly* 53, no. 211: 243–55.

Bourdieu, P. (1985). "The Forms of Capital." In J. G. Richardson, ed., *Handbook for Theory and Research for the Sociology of Education*, pp. 241–58. Westport, CT: Greenwood.

Bourdieu, P., and J-C. Passeron (1977/1990). *Reproduction in Education, Society and Culture*. London: Sage.

Breazeal, C. (2002). *Designing Social Robots*. Cambridge, MA: MIT Press.

Brooks, D. (2011). *The Social Animal*. New York: Random House.

Brothers, L. (1990). "The Social Brain: A Project for Integrating Primate Behavior and Neurophysiology in a New Domain." *Concepts in Neuroscience* 1: 27–51.

Brothers, L. (1997). *Friday's Footprint: How Society Shapes the Human Mind*. New York: Oxford University Press.

Brothers, L. (2001). *Mistaken Identity: The Mind-Brain Problem Reconsidered*. Albany: SUNY Press.

Brown, P. (1991). *The Hypnotic Brain: Hypnotherapy and Social Communication*. New Haven, CT: Yale University Press.

Bruce, K. D., A. Zsombok, and R. H. Eckel (2017). "Lipid Processing in the Brain: A Key Regulator of Systemic Metabolism." *Frontiers in Endocrinology* 8: 60.

Bruder, J. (2010). "The Brain, the Person, and the Social: How Can STS Deal with Neuroscience Objects and Practices?" *EASST Review*. https://www.easst.net/easst-review/easst-review-volume-294-december-2010/the-brain-the-person-and-the-social-how-can-sts-deal-with-neuroscience-objects-and-practices/.

Brueckner, A. (1986). "Brains in a Vat." Journal of Philosophy 83: 148–67.

Butler, J. (1993). *Bodies That Matter*. New York: Routledge.

Cacioppo, J., and W. Patrick (2008). *Loneliness: Human Nature and the Need for Social Connection*. New York: W. W. Norton.

Callaway, E. (2022). "Can Brain Scans Reveal Behavior? Bombshell Study Says Not Yet." *Nature* 603: 777.

Callero, P. L. (2013). *The Myth of Individualism: How Social Forces Shape Our Lives*. Lanham, MD: Rowman & Littlefield.

Campbell, D. T. (1960). "Blind Variation and Selective Retention in Creative Thought as in Other Knowledge Processes." *Psychological Review* 67: 380–400.

Cardenia, E. (2008). "Consciousness and Emotions as Interpersonal and Transpersonal Systems." In C. Whitehead, ed., *The Origins of Consciousness in the Social World*, pp. 249–63. Exeter: Imprint Academic.

Carhart-Harris, R. L., and K. J. Friston (2019). "REBUS and the Anarchic Brain: Toward a Unified Model of the Brain Action of Psychedelics." *Pharmacological Reviews* 71: 316–44.

Carr, C. J., and Z. Zukowski (2018). "Generating Albums with SampleRNN to Imitate Metal, Rock, and Punk Bands." *Proceedings of the Sixth International Workshop on Musical Metacreation*, arXiv:1811.06633v1[cs.SD].

Cattani, G. and S. Ferriani (2008). "A Core/Periphery Perspective on Individual Creative Performance: Social Networks and Cinematic Achievements in the Hollywood Film Industry." *Organization Science* 19, no. 6: 824–44.

Caves, R. (2000). *Creative Industries: Constructs Between Art and Commerce*. Cambridge, MA: Harvard University Press.

Chalmers, D. (2022a). "The Mind Bleeds into the World." *Edge*, October 29. https://www.edge.org/conversation/david_chalmers-the-mind-bleeds-into-the-world.

Chalmers, D. (2022b). *REALITY+: Virtual Worlds and the Problems of Philosophy*. New York: W. W. Norton.

Chang, L-C., J. Dattilo, and F-H. Huang (2022). "Relationships of Leisure Social Support and Flow with Loneliness in International Students in Taiwan: Implications during the COVID-19 Pandemic." *Leisure Sciences*. https://doi.org/10.1080/01490400.2022.2056550.

Clark, A. (1997). *Being There: Putting Brain, Body, and World Together Again*. Cambridge, MA: MIT Press.

Clark, A., and D. Chalmers (1998). "The Extended Mind." *Analysis* 58, no. 1: 7–19.

Cohen, A. P., and N. Rapport, eds. (1995). *Questions of Consciousness*. New York: Routlege.

Collins, R. (1973). *Conflict Sociology*. New York: Academic Press.

Collins, R. (1989). "Toward a Neo-Meadian Sociology of Mind." *Symbolic Interaction* 12: 1–32.

Collins, R. (1992). *Sociological Insight*. 2nd edition. Oxford: Oxford University Press.

Collins, R. (1998). *The Sociology of Philosophies*. Cambridge, MA: Harvard University Press.

Collins, R. (2004). *Interactional Ritual Chains*. Princeton, NJ: Princeton University Press.

Collins, R., and M. Makowsky (2010). *The Discovery of Society*. 8th edition. New York: McGraw Hill.

Colombo, J., et al. (2006). "Cerebral Cortex Astroglia and the Brain of a Genius: A Propos of A. Einstein." *Brain Research Reviews* 52, no. 2: 257–63.

Combs, A., and S. Krippner (2008). "Collective Consciousness and the Social Brain." In C. Whitehead, ed., *The Origins of Consciousness in the Social World*, pp. 264–76. Exeter: Imprint Academic.

Connolly, W. (2002). *Neuropolitics: Thinking, Culture, Speed*. Minneapolis: University of Minnesota Press.

Cooley, C. H. (1902). *Human Nature and the Social Order*. New York: Scribner's Sons.

Cooley, C. H. (1909). *Social Organization: A Study of the Larger Mind*. New York: Scriber's Sons.

Cozolino, L. (2012). *The Neuroscience of Psychotherapy: Healing the Social Brain*. Second edition. New York: Norton.

Crane, M. T. (2000). *Shakespeare's Brain*. Princeton, NJ: Princeton University Press.

Crick, F. C., and C. Koch (1990). "Towards a neurobiological theory of consciousness." *Seminars in the Neurosciences* 2: 263–275.

Csikszentmihalyi, M. (2008). *Flow: The Psychology of Optimal Experience*. New York: HarperCollins.

Csikszentmihalyi, M. (2014). *Applications of Flow in Human Development and Education, Collected Works*. New York: Springer.

Damasio, A. (1994). *Descartes' Error*. New York: G. P. Putnam.

Davis, J. E., and P. Scherz (2022). "Being Human in the Age of the Brain: Models of Mind and Their Social Effects." *Culture, Medicine, and Psychiatry* 46: 1–11.

Dawkins, R. (1976). *The Selfish Gene*. Oxford: Oxford University Press.

Dawkins, R. (2006). "It's All in the Genes." *The Sunday Times*, March 12.

de Lorenzo, V. (2018). "Evolutionary Tinkering vs. Rational Engineering in the Times of Synthetic Biology." *Life Sciences, Society and Policy* 14, no. 18: 1–16.

Dean, S. (2018). "The Human Brain Can Create Structures in Up to 11 Dimensions." ScienceAlert.com (summarizing Reimann, Nolte, et al. [2017]).

Decety, J., ed. (2020). *The Social Brain: A Developmental Perspective*. Cambridge, MA: MIT Press.

Dehaene, S. (2014). *Consciousness and the Brain: Deciphering How the Brain Codes Our Thoughts*. London: Penguin.

Deleuze, G., and F. Guattari (1987). *A Thousand Plateaus: Capitalism and Schizophrenia*. New York: Continuum.

Dennett, D. (2014). Intuition Pumps and Other Tools for Thinking. New York: W. W. Norton.

Denton, P. (2022). *The End of Technology*. Dubuque, IA: Kendall Hall.

DeSilva, J. M., J. F. A. Traniello, A. G Claxton, and L. D. Fannin (2021). "When and Why Did Human Brains Decrease in Size? A New Change-Point Analysis and Insights from Brain Evolution in Ants." *Frontiers in Ecology and Evolution* 9: 1–11.

DeVito, C. (2012). *Coltrane on Coltrane: The John Coltrane Interviews*. Chicago, IL: Chicago Review Press.

DeVore, B. (n.d.). "Primate Behavior and Social Evolution." Unpublished manuscript, cited in Geertz (1973, 68).

Diamond, J. (1998). *Guns, Germs, and Steel*. New York: W. W. Norton.

Dick, P. K. (2011). *Exegesis*. New York: Houghton, Mifflin, Harcourt.

Dominiak, S., et al. (2019). "Whisking Asymmetry Signals Motor Preparation and the Behavioral State of Mice." *Journal of Neuroscience* 39, no. 49: 9818–30.

Donald, M. (2001). *A Mind So Rare*. New York: W. W. Norton.

Doyle, R. (2004). "LSDNA: Consciousness Expansion and the Emergence of Biotechnology," pp. 103–120 in R. Mitchell and P. Thurtle, eds., *Data Made Flesh*. New York: Routledge.

Doyle, N. (2020). "Neurodiversity at Work: A Biopsychosocial Model and the Impact on Working Adults." *British Medical Bulletin* 135, no, 1: 108–25.

Dreyfus, H. L. (2007). "The Return of the Myth of the Mental." *Inquiry* 50, no. 4: 352–65.

Dumit, J. (2004). *Picturing Personhood: BrainScans and Biomedical Identity.* Princeton, NJ: Princeton University Press.

Dunbar, R. (1998). "The Social Brain Hypothesis." *Evolutionary Anthropology* 1, no. 8: 184–90.

Dunn, R. (2021). *A Natural History of the Future.* New York: Basic Books.

Durkheim, E. (1897/1952). *Suicide: A Study in Sociology.* London: Routledge and Kegan Paul.

Durkheim, E. (1912/1995). *The Elementary Forms of Religious Life.* New York: The Free Press.

Dyens, O. (2001). *Metal and Flesh: The Evolution of Man: Technology Takes Over.* Cambridge, MA: MIT Press.

Eagleman, D. (2015). *The Brain: The Story of You.* New York: Pantheon.

Epstein, R. (2021). "Your Brain Is Not a Computer. It Is a Transducer." *Discover*, August 25. https://www.discovermagazine.com/mind/your-brain-is-not-a-computer -it-is-a-transducer.

Erickson-Schroth, L. (2014). *Trans Bodies, Trans Selves: A Resource for the Transgender.* New York: Oxford University Press.

Espeso-Gil, S., et al., (2021). "Environmental Enrichment Induces Epigenomic and Genome Organization Changes Relevant for Cognition." *Frontiers in Molecular Neuroscience* 14: 1–19.

Farrell, M. (2001). *Collaborative Circles: Friendship Dynamics and Creative Work.* Chicago, IL: University of Chicago Press.

Farrera, A., and G. Ramos-Fernández (2022). "Rhythm as an Emergent Property during Human Social Coordination." *Frontiers in Psychology* 10. https://doi.org/10 .3389/fpsyg.2021.772262.

Faulkner, R. R. (2006). "Shedding Culture." In Becker et al., eds., *Art from Start to Finish*, pp. 91–117. Chicago, IL: University of Chicago Press.

Faulkner, R. R., and H. S. Becker (2009). *Do You Know . . . ? The Jazz Repertoire in Action.* Chicago, IL: University of Chicago Press.

Feynman, R. (1999). *The Pleasure of Finding Things Out.* New York: Basic Books.

Frank, L. (2009). *Mindfield: How Brain Science Is Changing Our World.* Oxford: Oneworld Publications.

Franks, D. (2019). *Neuroscience: Fundamentals and Current Findings.* New York: Springer.

Freeman, W. J., and G. Vitiello (2006). "Nonlinear brain dynamics and many-body field dynamics." *Electromagnetic Biology and Medicine* 24: 233–241.

Freud, S. (1895/1954). *The Origins of Psycho-Analysis: Letters to William Flies, Drafts and Notes 1887–1902.* New York: Basic Books.

Fries, P. (2005). "A mechanism for cognitive dynamics: neuronal communication through neuronal coherence." *Trends in Cognitive Science* 9: 474–480.

Fries, P. (2015). "Rhythms for cognition: communication through coherence," *Neuron* 88: 220–235.

Frith, C. D. (2008). "The Social Function of Consciousness." In L. Weiskrantz and M. Davies, eds., *Frontiers of Consciousness: Chichele Lectures*, pp. 225–44. Oxford: Oxford University Press.

Fuller, S. (2012). *Preparing for Life in Humanity 2.0*. New York: Palgrave PIVOT.

Gabora, L. (2013). "An Analysis of the 'Blind Variation and Selective Retention' Theory of Creativity." *Creativity Research Journal* 23, no. 2: 155–65.

Gabriel, E., M. Fenner, and J. Gopalakrishnan (2022). "Hirnorganoide entwickeln von Natur aus Augenprimordien." *BIOspektrum* 28, no. 5: 497–500.

Gao, H., J. R. Adrien, et al. (2017). "Overactivity of Liver-Related Neurons in the Paraventricular Nucleus of the Hypothalamus: Electrophysiological Findings." *Journal of Neuroscience* 37, no. 46: 11140–50.

Gardner, S. (2009). "Nietzsche, the Self, and the Disunity of Philosophical Reason." In K. Gemes and S. May, eds., *Nietzsche on Freedom and Autonomy*, pp. 1–31. Oxford: Oxford University Press.

Gaver, W. W. (1991). "Technology Affordances." In *Proceedings of the Human Factors in Computing Systems Conference*, pp. 79–84. New York: ACM Press.

Gaver, W. W. (1996). "Affordances for Interaction: The Social is Material for Design." *Ecological Psychology* 8, no. 2: 111–29.

Gazzaniga, M. (1985). *The Social Brain*. New York: Basic Books.

GCBH (Global Council on Brain Health) (2019). "The Real Deal on Brain Health Supplements: GCBH Recommendations on Vitamins, Minerals, and Other Dietary Supplements." www.GlobalCouncilOnBrainHealth.org.

Geertz, C. (1973). *The Interpretation of Cultures*. New York: Basic Books.

Geertz, C. (2000). *Available Light: Anthropological Reflections on Philosophical Topics*. Princeton, NJ: Princeton University Press.

Gemes, K., and S. May, eds. (2009). *Nietzsche on Freedom and Autonomy*. New York: Oxford University Press.

Gibson, J. J. (1966). *The Senses Considered as Perceptual Systems*. Westport, CT: Greenwood Press.

Gibson, W. (1984). *Neuromancer*. New York: ACE.

Giurgea, C. (1972). "Pharmacology of integrative Activity of the Brain: Attempt at Nootropic Concept in Psychopharmacology." *Actualites Pharmacologiques* 25: 115–56.

Giurgea, C., and M. Salama (1977). "Nootropic Drugs." *Progress in Neuro-Psychopharmacology* 1, nos. 3–4: 235–47.

Goffman, E. (1959). *The Presentation of Self in Everyday Life*. New York: Anchor Books.

Goffman, E. (1974). *Frame Analysis: An Essay on the Organization of Experience*. Cambridge, MA: Harvard University Press.

Goffman, E. (1982). *Interaction Ritual*. New York: Pantheon.

Goldstein, D. B., et al. (2003). "Pharmacogenetics Goes Genomic." *Nature Reviews Genetics* 4: 937–47.

Gordon, A., et al. (2021). "Long-Term Maturation of Human Cortical Organoids Matches Key Early Postnatal Transitions." *Nature Neuroscience* 24, no. 3: 331–42.

Gorney, R. (1972). *The Human Agenda*. New York: Bantam.

Gotman, K. (2012). The Neural Metaphor." In M. M. Littlefield and J. M. Johnson, eds., *The Neuroscience Turn: Transdisciplinarity in the Age of the Brain*, pp. 71–80. Ann Arbor: University of Michigan Press.

Gottlieb, G. (2007). "Probabilistic Epigenesis." *Developmental Science* 10, no. 1: 1–1.

Grand View Research (2022). *Brain Health Supplements Market Size, Share and Trends Analysis Report by Product (Natural Molecules, Herbal Extract), by Application, by Region, and Segment Forecasts, 2020–2030.*

Granovetter, M. (1973). "The Strength of Weak Ties." *American Journal of Sociology* 78, no. 6: 1360–80.

Graziano, M. S. A. (2013). *Consciousness and the Social Brain.* Oxford: Oxford University Press.

Grossberg, S. (2017). "Towards solving the hard problem of consciousness: the varieties of brain resonances and the conscious experiences that they support." *Neural Networks* 87: 38–95.

Haga, S. B., and W. Burke (2004). "Using Pharmacogenetics to Improve Drug Safety and Efficacy." *Journal of the American Medical Association* 291: 2869–71.

Hagmann, P. (2005). *From Diffusion MRI to Brain Connectomics.* PhD Dissertation, Polytechnique Fédérale de Lausanne.

Haldane, J. B. S. (1924). *Daedalus, or The Future of Science.* New York: E. P. Dutton.

Hanalioglu, S., et al. (2021). "Group-Level Ranking-Based Hubness Analysis of Human Brain Connectome Reveals Significant Interhemispheric Asymmetry and Intraparcel Heterogeneities." *Frontiers in Neuroscience* 21: 1–14.

Hanh, T. N., and N. Anh-Huong (2006). *Walking Meditation.* Boulder, CO: Sounds True Publishing.

Hansen, M. (2015). *Feed Forward.* Chicago, IL: University of Chicago Press.

Hantel, M. (2020). "Plasticity and Fungibility: On Sylvia Wynter's Pieza Framework." *Social Text* 38, no. 2: 97–119.

Harman, G. (1973/2016). *Thought.* Princeton, NJ: Princeton University Press.

Harper, G. W., J. Davidson, and S. G. Hosek (2008). "Influence of Gang Membership on Negative Affect, Substance Use, and Antisocial Behavior Among Homeless African American Male Youth." *American Journal of Men's Health* 2, no. 3: 229–43.

Harvard Health Publishing (2022). "Don't Buy into Brain Health Supplements."

Hayden, T. (1967). "A Letter to the New (Young) Left." In M. Cohen and D. Hale, eds., *The New Student Left*, revised and expanded edition, pp. 2–9. Boston: Beacon Press.

Hayes, N. (2018). *Your Brain and You: A Simple Guide to Neuropsychology.* London: TeachYourself.

Hayles, K. (1999). *How We Became Posthuman: Virtual Bodies in Cybernetics, Literature, and Information.* Chicago: University of Chicago Press.

Hayles, K. (2004). "Flesh and Metal: Reconfiguring the Mindbody," pp. 229–48 in R. Mitchell and P. Thurtle, eds., *Data Made Flesh.* New York: Routledge.

Heckathorn, D., and J. Jeffri (2001). "Finding the Beat: Using Respondent-Driven Sampling to Study Jazz Musicians." *Poetics* 28: 307–29.

Heckathorn, D., and J. Jeffri (2003). "Social Networks of Jazz Musicians." In *Changing the Beat: A Study of the Worklife of Jazz Musicians, Volume III: Respondent-Driven Sampling: Survey Results by the Research Center for Arts and*

Culture, pp. 48–61. National Endowment for the Arts Research Division Report #43. Washington, DC.

Heimerdinger, M., and A. LaViers (2019). "Modeling the Interactions of Context and Style on Affect in Motion Perception: Stylized Gaits Across Multiple Environmental Contexts." *International Journal of Social Robotics* 11, no 3: 495–513.

Henrich, J. (2008). "A Cultural Species: Why a Theory of Culture Required to Build a Science of Human Behavior." https://henrich.fas.harvard.edu/files/henrich/files/henrich_2008–2.pdf.

Hentsch, T. (2004). *Truth or Death: The Quest for Immortality in the Western Narrative Tradition*. Vancouver, BC: Talonbooks.

Highfield, R., and P. Carter (1993). *The Private Lives of Albert Einstein*. New York: St. Martin's Press.

Hood, B. (2012). *The Self Illusion: How the Social Brain Creates Identity*. New York: Oxford University Press.

Horowitz, S. (2010). "Health Benefits of Meditation: What the Newest Research Shows." *Alternative and Complementary Therapies* 16, no. 4: 223–28.

Hossenfelder, S. (2022). *Existential Physics*. New York: Viking.

Hu, P., J. Park, and A. Roskies (2021). "What Is the Readiness Potential?" *Trends in Cognitive Science* 25, no. 7: 558–70.

Hunt, T., and J. W. Schooler (2019). "The Easy Part of the Hard Problem: A Resonance Theory of Consciousness." *Frontiers of Human Neuroscience* 31: 1–16.

Irvine, T., and V. Cardo (2019–2021). "Jazz as Social Machine: Investigating the Human Complexities at the Border Between AI and Jazz Improvisation." https://www.turing.ac.uk/research/research-projects/jazz-social-machine.

Jacob, F. (1977). "Evolution and Tinkering." *Science* 196, no. 4295: 1161–66.

Jacobs, G. (2006). *Charles Horton Cooley: Imagining Social Reality*. Amherst: University of Massachusetts Press.

Jaeggi, R. (2014). *Alienation*. New York: Columbia University Press.

Jordania, J. (2011). *Why Do People Sing? Music in Human Evolution*. Tbilisi, Georgia: Logos.

Joyce, K. (2008). *Magnetic Appeal: MRI and the Myth of Transparency*. Ithaca, NY: Cornell University Press.

Kapferer, B. (1995). "From the Edge of Death: Sorcery and the Motion of Consciousness." In A. P. Cohen and N. Rapport, eds., *Questions of Consciousness*, pp. 134–52. New York: Routledge.

Kaptelinin, V. (2014). *Affordances and Design*. Aarhus, Denmark: The Interaction Design Foundation.

Karatani, K. (2003). *Transcritique*. Cambridge, MA: MIT Press.

Karzal, A. (2019). *Nietzsche and Sociology: Prophet of Affirmation*. Lanham, MD: Lexington Books.

Keller, E. F. (1983). *A Feeling for the Organism: The Life and Work of Barbara McClintock*. New York: W. H. Freeman.

Keller, P. E., G. Novembre, and M. J. Hove (2014). "Rhythm in Joint Action: Psychological and Neurophysiological Mechanisms for Real-Time Interpersonal Coordination." *Philosophical Transactions of the Royal Society,* London, B,

Biological Sciences, 369 (1658). https://www.ncbi.nlm.nih.gov/pmc/articles/
PMC424097/.

Kelly, K. (2012). *What Technology Wants*. New York: Viking.

Khanna, P. (2016). *Connectography: Mapping the Future of Global Civilization*. New York: Random House.

Kirschbaum, C., and P. F. Ribeiro (2016). "How Social Network Role, Geographical Context and Territorial Mobility Mediate the Adoption of Transgressive Styles in the Jazz Field." *Journal of Economic Geography* 16: 1187–1210.

Knorr-Cetina, K. (1979). "Tinkering Toward Success." *Theory and Society* 8: 347–76.

Koch, C. (2004). *The Quest for Consciousness: A Neurobiological Approach*. Boston: Roberts Publishers.

Kong, L. (2022). "The Search for Immortality." *History Today* 72, no. 4. https://www.historytoday.com/archive/history-matters/search-immortality.

Kornhuber H. H., and L. Deecke (1965). "Hirnpotentialänderungen bei Willkürbewegungen und passiven Bewegungen des Menschen: Bereitschaftspotential und reafferente Potentiale." *Pflügers Arch.* 284: 1–17.

Kroeber, A. (1963). *Configurations of Culture Growth*. Berkeley: University of California Press.

Kropotkin, P. (1908). *Modern Science and Anarchism*. New York: Mother Earth Publishing.

Krubitzer, L. (2014). "Lessons from Evolution." In G. Marcus and J. Freeman, eds., *The Future of the Brain: Essays by the World's Leading Neuroscientists*, pp. 186–93. Princeton, NJ: Princeton University Press.

Kruger, J., and D. Dunning (2000). "Unskilled and Unaware of It: How Difficulties in Recognizing One's Own Incompetence Lead to Inflated Self-Assessments." *Journal of Personality and Social Psychology* 77, no. 6: 1121–34.

Lahav, N., and Z. A. Neemeh (2022). "A Relativistic Theory of Consciousness: Hypothesis and Theory." *Frontiers in Psychology* (May 12): 1–25.

Langer, E. J., A. Blank and B. Chanowitz (1978). "The Mindlessness of Ostensibly Thoughtful Action: The Role of 'Placebic' Information In Interpersonal Interaction." *Journal of Personality and Social Psychology* 36, no. 6: 635–42.

LaViers, A., Y. Chen, C. Belta, and M. Egerstedt (2011). "Automatic Sequencing of Ballet Poses: A Formal Approach to Phrase Generation." *IEEE Robotics and Automation Magazine* (September): 87–95.

LaViers, A., C. Cuan, C. Maguire, K. Bradley, K. Brooks Mata, A. Nilles, I. Vidrin, N. Chakraborty, M. Heimerdinger, U. Huzaifa, R. McNish, I. Pakrasi, and A. Zurawski (2018). "Choreographic and Somatic Approaches for the Development of Expressive Robotic Systems." *Arts MDPI* (Special Issue on Machine as Artist for the 21st Century).

Lehmertz, K., C. E. Elger, J. Arnold, and P. Grassberger, eds. (2000). "Workshop on Chaos in Brain." *Proceedings of the 1999 Workshop*. Singapore: World Scientific.

Lemert, C., ed. (2021). *Social Theory: The Multicultural, Global, and Classic Readings*. 7th edition. New York: Routledge.

Levi-Strauss, C. (1967). *The Savage Mind*. Chicago: University of Chicago Press.

Lewis, C. S. (1990). *Studies in Words*. Cambridge, UK: Cambridge University Press.

Li, J-Z, et al. (2021). "An Enriched Environment Delays the Progression from Mild Cognitive Impairment to Alzheimer's Disease in Senescence Accelerated Mouse Prone 8 Mice." *Experimental and Therapeutic Medicine* 22, 5: 1–12.

Libet, B. (1985). "Unconscious Cerebral Initiative and the Role of Conscious Will in Voluntary Action." *The Behavioral and Brain Sciences* 8, no. 4: 529–66.

Lieberman, M. D. (2013). *Social: Why Our Brains Are Wired to Connect*. New York: Crown Publishers.

Limb, C., and M. López-González (2012). "Musical Creativity and the Brain." *Cerebrum* 3, no. 2. Published online February 22, 2012.

Littlefield, M. M., and J.M. Johnson, eds. (2012). *The Neuroscience Turn: Transdisciplinarity in the Age of the Brain*. Ann Arbor: University of Michigan Press.

Lopez, R. (2010). "Welcome to Your Social Brain." *Psychology Today*, July 11. https://www.psychologytoday.com/us/blog/our-social-brains/201007/welcome -your-social-brain.

Luo, C., et al. (2016). "Cerebral Organoids Recapitulate Epigenomic Signatures of the Human Fetal Brain." *Cell Reports* 17, no. 12: 3369–84.

Lycan, W. (1996). *Consciousness and Experience*. Cambridge, MA: MIT Press.

Macfarlane, A. (2019). "Gangs and Adolescent Mental Health: A Narrative Review." *Journal of Child and Adolescent Trauma* 12, no. 3: 411–20.

Mackenzie, R. (2022). "Stats Study Reveals Reason for Replication Crisis in Neuroscience." *Technology Networks Neuroscience News and Research*, March 16.

Mahfoud, T. (2014). "Extending the Mind: A Review of Ethnographies of Neuroscience Practice." *Frontiers of Human Neuroscience* 8, no. 359: 1–9.

Marek, S., B. Tenyo-Clemmens, and N. U. F. Dosenbach (2022). "Reproducible Brain-Wide Association Studies Require Thousands of Individuals." *Nature* 603: 654–60.

Marino, T., C. Widdowson, A. Oetting, A. Lakshmanan, H. Cui, N. Hovakimyan, R. Wang, A. Kirlik, A. LaViers, D. Stipanovic (2016). "Carebots: Prolonged Elderly Independence Using Small Mobile Robots." *Mechanical Engineering* 138, no. 9: S8.

Markram, H. (2008). "Fixing the Location and Dimensions of Functional Neocortical Columns." *Human Frontiers Science Program Journal* 3: 132–35.

Martin, E. (1992). "The End of the Body?" in *American Ethnologist* 19, no. 1: 121–40.

Martino, A. (2022). "Salman Rushdie and the Freedom to Offend." http://www .worldliteraturetoday.org.

Marx, K. (1844/1956). *The Economic and Philosophic Manuscripts of 1844.* Moscow: Foreign Languages Publishing House.

Marx, K. (1847/1957). "Contribution to the Critique of Hegel's Philosophy of Right." In K. Marx and F. Engels, *On Religion*, pp. 41–58. Moscow: Foreign Languages Publishing House.

Marx, K. (1857–1858/1973). *The Grundrisse* (unfinished manuscript). New York: Harper & Row.

Marx, K., and F. Engels (1932/2004). *The German Ideology*. New York: International Publishers (originally written 1845–1848).

Maryanski, A. (2018). *Emile Durkheim and the Birth of the Gods*. New York: Routledge.

Masterson, V. (2022). "This Could Be a Simple Solution to Loneliness, According to Scientists." *World Economic Forum*, April 15. https://europeansting.com/2022/04/15/this-could-be-a-simple-solution-to-loneliness-according-to-scientists/.

McAndrew, S., P. Widdop, and R. Stevenson (2015). "On Jazz Worlds," in N. Crossley, S. McAndrew, and P. Widdop, eds., *Social Networks and Music Worlds*, pp. 217–43. New York: Routledge.

McCraty, R. (2015). *Science of the Heart: Exploring the Role of the Heart in Human Performance.* Volume 2. Boulder Creek, CA: HeartMath Institute.

McNeill, W. H. (1963). *The Rise of the West*. Chicago, IL: University of Chicago Press.

Mead, G. H. (1934). *Mind, Self and Society*. Chicago, IL: University of Chicago Press.

Mele, A. (2014). *Why Science Hasn't Disproved Free Will*. New York: Oxford University Press.

Mele, A. (2017). *Aspects of Agency: Decisions, Abilities, Explanations, and Free Will*. New York: Oxford University Press.

Menger, P-M. (2006). "Profiles of the Unfinished: Rodin's Work and the Varieties of Incompleteness."In Becker, et al., eds., *Art from Start to Finish*, pp. 31–68. Chicago, IL: University of Chicago Press.

Mercier, H., and D. Sperber (2017). *The Enigma of Reason*. Cambridge, MA: Harvard University Press.

Merton, R. K. (1961). "Singletons and Multiples in Scientific Discovery: A Chapter in the Sociology of Science." *Proceedings of the American Philosophical Society* 105: 470–86; reprinted in R. K. Merton (1973), *The Sociology of Science* (Chicago, IL: University of Chicago Press), 343–70.

Merton, R. K. (1965). *Standing on the Shoulders of Giants: A Shandean Postscript*. Chicago, IL: University of Chicago Press.

Mialet, H. (2012). *Hawking Incorporated: Stephen Hawking and the Anthropology of the Knowing Subject*. Chicago, IL: University of Chicago Press.

Mills, C. W. (1939). "Language, Logic and Culture." *American Sociological Review* 4, no. 5: 670–80; reprinted in Mills (1963: 423–38).

Mills, C. W. (1959). *The Sociological Imagination*. Oxford: Oxford University Press.

Mills, C. W. (1963). "Language. Logic, and Culture." In I. L. Horowitz, ed., *Power, Politics, and People*, pp. 423–38. New York: Ballantine Books.

Milton, J. (1674/2013). *John Milton: Paradise Lost*. New York: Palgrave Macmillan.

Mitchell, R. (2004). "Sell: Body Wastes, Information, and Commodification," pp. 121–36 in R. Mitchell and P. Thurtle, eds., *Data Made Flesh*. New York: Routledge.

Mithen, S. J. (2005). *The Singing Neanderthals: The Origins of Music, Language, Mind and Body*. Cambridge, MA: Harvard University Press.

Mohammed, A. H., et al., (2002). "Enviromental Enrichment and the Brain." *Progress in Brain Research* 138: 109–33.

Montagu, A. (1952). *Darwin, Competition, and Cooperation*. New York: Henry Schuman.

Montagu, A. (1971). *Touching: The Human Significance of the Skin*. New York: Harper and Row.

Moore, D. (2001). *The Dependent Gene*. New York: Henry Holt.

Morana, A. (2008). "Working with Brain Scans: Digital Images and Gestural Interactionin fMRI Laboratory." *Social Studies of Science* 38: 483–508.

Moravec, H. (1999). "Simulation, Consciousness, Existence." *Intercommunications* 28: 98–112.

Morison, J. S. (2012). "'The Paradise of Non-Experts': The Neuroscientific Turn of the 1840s United States." In M. M. Littlefield and J. M. Johnson, eds., *The Neuroscience Turn: Transdisciplinarity in the Age of the Brain*, pp. 29–48. Ann Arbor: University of Michigan Press.

Neuhouser, F., and A. E. Smith (2018). "Alienation." *Stanford Encyclopedia of Philosophy*. Stanford, CA: Stanford University Press.

Newcomb, T. (1943). *Personality and Social Change: Attitude Formation in a Student Community*. New York: Dryden.

Newcomb, T., K. E. Koenig, R. Flacks, and D. P. Warwick (1967). *Persistence and Change: Bennington College and Its Students after 25 Years*. New York: Wiley.

Nicolelis, M. (2011). *Beyond Boundaries*. New York: Henry Holt and Co.

Nietzsche, F. (1878/1996). *Human, All Too Human*. Cambridge, UK: Cambridge University Press.

Nietzsche, F. (1881/2007). *The Dawn of the Day*. Mineola, NY: Dover.

Nietzsche, F. (1886/1989). *Beyond Good and Evil*. New York: Vintage.

Nietzsche, F. (1887). *Die fröhliche Wissenschaft*. Leipzig, Germany: W. W. Fritsch.

Nietzsche, F. (1887/1994). *On the Genealogy of Morals*. Cambridge, UK: Cambridge University Press.

Nietzsche, F. (1887/1974). *The Gay Science*. New York: Vintage.

Nietzsche, F. (1889, 1895/1968). *Twilight of the Idols/The Anti-Christ*. New York: Penguin.

Nietzsche, F. (1888/1992). *Ecce Homo*. New York: Penguin.

Nightline (2002). ABC-TV, August 19: Discussion of socially competent robots.

Noble, S., A. F. Meija, A. Zalesky, and D. Scheinost (2022). "Improving Power in Functional Magnetic Resonance Imaging by Moving Beyond Cluster-Level Inference." *Proceedings of the National Academy of Sciences* 119, no. 32: 1–10.

Noë, A. (2009). *Out of Our Heads: Why You Are Not Your Brain, and Other Lessons from the Biology of Consciousness*. NewYork: Hill & Wang.

Noorani, T., and B. A. Day (2020). "Spotlight Commentary: REBUS and the Anarchic Brain." *Neuroscience of Consciousness* 1: 1–3.

Norman, D. (1988). *The Psychology of Everyday Things*. New York: Basic Books.

O'Hare, J. D., and A. Zsombok (2016). *American Journal of Physiological Endocrinology Metabolism* 310, no. 3: E183–89.

Okruszek, Ł., et al. (2021). "Owner of a Lonely Mind? Social cognitive Capacity Is Associated with Objective, But Not Perceived Social Isolation in Healthy

Individuals." *Journal of Research in Personality* 93. https://doi.org/10.1016/j.jrp .2021.104103.

Onaolapo, A. Y., A. Y. Oelawo, and O. J. Onaolapo (2019). "Brain Ageing, Cognition and Diet: A Review of the Emerging Roles of Food-Based Nootropics in Mitigating Age-Related Memory Decline." *Current Aging Science* 12, 1: 2–14.

Pascal. B. (1670/1995). *The Pensée*. New York: Penguin.

Penrose, R. (1989). *The Emperor's New Mind*. New York: Oxford University Press.

Penrose, R., and S. R. Hameroff (1995). "What Gaps? Reply to Grush and Churchland." *Journal of Consciousnesss Studies* 2: 99–112.

Pert, C. (1997). *Molecules of Emotion*. New York: Scribner.

Perry, J. (2004). "Jazz and Innovation: How the Jazz Culture Fosters Creativity." *All About Jazz*, February 10.

Pescosolido, B. A. (2011). "Organizing the Sociological Landscape for the Next Decades of Health and Health Care Research: The Network Episode Model III-R as Cartographic Subfield Guide." In B. A. Pescosolido, J. K. Martin, J. D. McLeod, and A. Rogers, eds., *Handbook of the Sociology of Health, Illness, and Healing*, pp. 39–66. New York: Springer.

Phillips-Silver, J., C. A. Aktipis, and G. A. Bryant (2010). "The Ecology of Entrainment: Foundations of Coordinated Rhythmic Movement." *Music Perception* 28, no. 1: 3–14.

Pickersgill, M. (2013). "The Social Life of the Brain: Neuroscience in Society." *Current Sociology* 61, no. 3: 322–40.

Pickersgill, M., and I. Van Keulen, eds. (2012). *Sociological Reflections on the Neurosciences*. Bingley, UK: Emerald.

Pitts-Taylor, V. (2016). *The Brain's Body*. Durham NC: Duke University Press.

Pockett, S. (2000). *The Nature of Consciousness.* San Jose, CA: Writers Club Press.

Pockett, S. (2012). "The electromagnetic field theory of consciousness: a testable hypothesis about the characteristics of conscious as opposed to non-conscious fields." *Journal of Consciousness Studies* 19: 191–203.

Porter, J. (2015). *The Vertical Mosaic: An Analysis of Social Class and Power in Canada*. 50th anniversary edition. Toronto: University of Toronto Press.

Porter, L. (1999). *John Coltrane: His Life and Music*. Ann Arbor: University of Michigan Press.

Poster, M. (2004). "Desiring Information and Machines," pp. 87–102 in R. Mitchell and P. Thurtle, eds., *Data Made Flesh*. New York: Routledge.

Purvis, K. (2016). *Theology and the University in Nineteenth-Century Germany*. Oxford: Oxford University Press.

Putnam, H. (1981). *Reason, Truth, and History*. Cambridge, UK: Cambridge University Press.

Putnam, R. (2000). *Bowling Alone*. New York: Simon & Schuster.

Ratliff, B. (2007). *Coltrane: The Story of a Sound*. London: Faber & Faber.

Rapp, R. (2011). "Chasing science: children's brains, scientific inquiries, andfamily Labors." *Science, Technology and Human Values* 36: 662–84.

Reardon. S. (2020). "Can Lab-Grown Brains Become Conscious." *Nature* 576: 658–61.

Reimann, M., et al. (2017). "Cliques of Neurons Bound into Cavities Provide a Missing Link Between Structure and Function." *Frontiers in Computational Neuroscience* 11, no. 48: 1–16.

Restak, R. (2006). *The Naked Brain: How the Emerging Neurosociety Is Changing How We Live, Work, and Love.* New York: Crown.

Restivo, S. (2011). "Bruno Latour: The Once and Future Philosopher," pp. 520–40 in G. Ritzer and J. Stepinsky, eds., *The New Blackwell Companion to Major Social Theorists.* Boston: Blackwell.

Restivo, S. (2017). *Sociology, Science, and the End of Philosophy: How Society Shapes Brains, Gods, Maths, and Logics.* New York: Palgrave Macmillan).

Restivo, S. (2018). *The Age of the Social.* New York: Routledge.

Restivo, S. (2020). *Einstein's Brain: Genius, Culture, and Social Networks.* New York: Palgrave Pivot.

Restivo, S. (2021). *Society and the Death of God.* New York: Routledge.

Restivo, S. (2022). *Inventions in Sociology: Studies in Science and Society.* New York: Palgrave Macmillan.

Restivo, S. (2023). *Beyond the New Atheism and Theism: A Sociology of Science, Secularism, and Religiosity.* New York: Routledge.

Restivo, S., and A. Steinhauer (2000). "Toward a Socio-Visual Theory of Information and Information Technology." Paper presented at the IEEE International Symposium on Technology and Society, Department of Electronic Engineering, La Sapienza University, Rome, IT, September.

Restivo, S., M. Incayawar, and J. M. Clarke (2020). "The Social Brain: Implications for Therapeutic and Preventive Protocols in Psychiatry." In S. Restivo, *Einstein's Brain*, pp. 123–37. New York: Palgrave Pivot.

Restivo, S., and J. Loughlin (2000). "The Invention of Science." *Cultural Dynamics* 12, no. 2: 135–49.

Restivo, S., S. Weiss, and A. Stingl (2014). *Worlds of ScienceCraft.* New York: Routledge.

Ricci, G. (2020). "Pharmacological Human Enhancement: An Overview of the Looming Bioethical and Regulatory Challenges." *Frontiers in Psychiatry* 11: 1–6. https://www.frontiersin.org/articles/10.3389/fpsyt.2020.00053/full.

Richards, P., and G. Ruivenkamp (1996). "New Tools for Conviviality: Society and Biotechnology." In P. Descola and G. Palsson, eds., *Nature and Society: Anthropological Perspectives*, pp. 275–95. New York: Routledge.

Ridley, M. (2008). *The Cooperative Gene.* New York: The Free Press.

Rigoni, D., S. Kuhn, G. Sartori, and M. Brass (2011). "Inducing Disbelief in Free Will Alters Brain Correlates of Preconscious Motor Preparation: The Brain Minds Whether We Believe in Free Will or Not." *Psychological Science* 22, no. 5: 613–28.

Rose, H., and S. Rose (2016). *Can Neuroscience Change Our Minds?* Cambridge: Polity.

Rose, N., and J. M. Abi-Rached (2013). *Neuro: The New Brain Sciences and the Management of the Mind.* Princeton, NJ: Princeton University Press.

Rose, S. (2005). *The Future of the Brain.* Oxford: Oxford University Press.

Rosen, D. S., Y. Oh, B. Erickson, F. Z. Youngmoo, E. Kim, and J. Kounios (2020). "Dual-Process Contributions to Creativity in Jazz Improvisations: An SPM-EEG Study." *Neuroimage* 213: 1–12.

Rosenberg, L. (2022). "Identity Crisis: Artificial Intelligence and the Flawed Logic of 'Mind Uploading.'" *VentureBeat*, August 13.

Roser, M. E., and M. S. Gazzaniga (2009). "Split-Brain Patients." In L. R. Squire, ed., *Encyclopedia of Neuroscience*, pp. 351–56. London: Academic Press.

Roszak, T. (1986). *The Cult of Information*. Berkeley: University of California Press.

Roth, M. E., J. M. Gillis, and F. D. DiGennaro Reed (2014). "A MetaAnalysis of Behavioral Interventions for Adolescents and Adults with Autism Spectrum Disorders." *Journal of Behavioral Education* 23: 258–86.

Roughgarden, J. (2009). *Le Géne Généreux*. Berkeley: University of California Press.

Russell, B. (1924). *Icarus, The Future of Science*. New York: E. P. Dutton.

Ryle, G. (1949). *The Concept of Mind*. Chicago, IL: University of Chicago Press.

Sahu, S., S. Ghosh, B. Ghosh, K. Aswani, et al. (2013). "Atomic water channel controlling remarkable properties of a single brain microtubule: Correlating single protein to its supramolecular assembly." *Biosensors and Bioelectronics* 2013: 141–148.

Sahu, S., S. Ghosh, K. Hirata, D. Fujita, and A. Bandyopadhyay (2013). "Multi-level Memory-switching Properties of a Single Brain Microtubule," *Applied Physical Letters* 2013: 123701.

Sanderson, B. (2015). *Perfect State*. American Fort, UT: Dragonsteel Entertainment.

Sawyer, K. (2008). *Group Genius: The Creative Power of Collaboration*. New York: Basic Books.

Scalzi, J. (2005). *Old Man's War*. New York: Tor Books.

Seabrook, J. (1993). "Biotechnology and Genetic Diversity." *Race and Class* 34, no. 3: 15–30.

Searle, J. (1992). *The Rediscovery of Mind.* Cambridge, MA: MIT Press.

Shapson-Coe, A., et al. (2021). "A Connectomic Study of a Petascale Fragment of Human Cerebral Cortex." *BioR_xiv*: 1–95.

Shelley, M. (1831/1994). *Frankenstein*. New York: Dover.

Siegel, D. J., and T. P. Bryson (2012). *The Whole-Brain Child*. New York: Bantam.

Simonton, D. K. (1999). *Origins of Genius*. New York: Oxford University Press.

Simonton, D. K. (2012). "Creative Thought as Blind Variation and Selective Retention: Why Creativity Is Inversely Related to Sightedness." *Journal of Theoretical and Philosophical Psychology* 33, no. 4: 253–66.

Singh, P., K. Ray, D. Fujita, and A. Bandyopadhyay (2018). "Complete Dielectric Resonator Model of Human Brain from MRI Data: A Journey from Connectome Neural Branching to Single Protein." *Engineering Vibration, Communication and Information Processing* 478: 717–733.

Skarda, C. A., and W. J. Freeman (1987). "How Brains Make Chaos in Order to Make Sense of the World." *Behavioral and Brain Sciences* 10: 161–95.

Skarda, C. A., and W. J. Freeman (1990). "Chaos and the New Science of the Brain." *Concepts in Neuroscience* 2: 275–85.

Slaby, J., and S. Gallagher (2014). "Critical Neuroscience and Socially Extended Minds." *Theory, Culture, and Society* 6, no. 11: 1–27.

Smith, A. (1759/2012). *The Theory of Moral Sentiments*. London: Penguin Classics.

Soegaard, M. (2015). "Affordances." In B. Papantoniou et al., eds., *Glossary of Human Computer Interaction*. Aarhus, Denmark: The Interaction Design Foundation.

Soresi, E. (2005). *Il Cervello Anarchico*. Torino, Italy: UTET.

Southern, S. (1989). "Consciousness." *Macmillan Dictionary of Psychology*. New York: Macmillan.

Sporns, O. G., G. Tononi, and R. Kötter (2005). "The Human Connectome: A Structural Description of the Human Brain." *PLoS Computational Biology* 1, no. 4: c42.

Stam, C. J. (2005). "Nonlinear Dynamical Analysis of EEG and MEG: Review of an Emerging Field." *Clinical Neurophysiology* 116: 2266–301.

Star, S. L. (1989). *Regions of the Mind: Brain Research and the Quest for Scientific Certainty*. Stanford, CA: Stanford University Press.

Star, S. L., and J. Griesemer (1989). "Institutional Ecology, 'Translations' and Boundary Objects: Amateurs and Professionals in Berkeley's Museum of Vertebrate Zoology, 1907–39." *Social Studies of Science* 19, no. 3: 387–420.

Stoltz, S. (2020). "Nietzsche's Psychology of the Self: The Art of Overcoming the Divided Self." *Human Arenas* 3, no. 2: 264–78.

Stone, M. H. (1997). *Healing the Mind: A History of Psychiatry from Antiquity to the Present*. New York: W. W. Norton.

Strathern, M. (1992). *Reproducing the Future: Anthropology, Knowledge and the New Reproductive Technologies*. Manchester, UK: Manchester University Press.

Sutherland S. (1989). *The International Dictionary of Psychology*. New York: Crossroads Classic.

Sydie, R. A. (1987). *Natural Women/Cultured Men*. London: Metheun.

Sykes, R. W. (2020). *Kindred*. New York: Bloomsbury Sigma.

Swart, T., K. Chisholm, and P. Brown (2015). *Neuroscience for Leadership: Harnessing the Brain Gain Advantage*. New York: Palgrave Macmillan.

Takatoh, J., et al. (2022). "The Whisking Oscillator Circuit." *Nature*. https://doi.org/10.1038/s41586-022-05144-8.

Taylor, S. (2012). *Back to Sanity*. London: Hay House.

Teitelbaum, T., P. Balenzuela, P. Cano, and J. M. Buldu (2008). "Community Structures and Role Detection in Music Networks." *Chaos* 18, no. 043105. https://doi.org/10.1063/1.2988285.

TenHouten, W. (1997). "Neurosociology." *Journal of Social and Evolutionary Systems* 20, no. 1: 7–37.

Thomas, M. (2022). What Is Simulation Theory? Are We Living in a Computer Simulation?" *Built In*. https://builtin.com/hardware/simulation-theory.

Thomas, P. (1985). *Karl Marx and the Anarchists*. London: Routledge and Kegan Paul.

Thorpe, C. (2020). "Book Review: A. Karzal, Nietzsche and Sociology (2019)." *European Journal of Social Theory* 23, no. 1: 113–18.

Tolstoy, L. (1869/1996). *War and Peace*. New York: W. W. Norton.

Torrance, S., and F. Schumann (2019). "The Spur of the Moment: What Jazz Improvisation Tells Cognitive Science." *AI & Society* 34: 251–68.

Trevarthen, C. (1979). "Communication and Cooperation in Early Infancy: A Description of Primary Intersubjectivity." In M. Bullowa, ed., *Before Speech: The Beginnings of Human Communication*, pp. 321–47. Cambridge, UK: Cambridge University Press.

Turner, R. (2002). "Culture and the Human Brain." *Anthropology and Humanism* 26: 1–6.

Turner, R., and Whitehead, C. (2008). "How collective Representations Can Change the Structure of the Brain." *Journal of Consciousness Studies* 15: 43–57.

Turner, S. (2002). *Brains/Practices/Relativism: Social Theory after Cognitive Science*. Chicago, IL: University of Chicago Press.

Turner, S. (2018). *Cognitive Science and the Social*. New York: Routledge.

Turner, V. (1982). *From Ritual to Theatre: The Human Seriousness of Play*. New York: Performing Arts Journal Publications.

Ulbach, L. (1860). "Le Prince Bonifacio." In *L'Isle des Rêves*. Paris: Morizot, Libraire-Editeur.

Umberson, D., and J. K. Montez (2010). "Social Relationships and Health: A Flashpoint for Health Policy." *Journal of Health and Social Behavior* 51 (Suppl.): S54–S66.

Underwood, E. (2021). "Newly Detailed Nerve Links Between Brain and Other Organs Shape Thoughts, Memories, and Feelings." *Brain & Behavior*. https://doi .org/10.1126/science.abb3221.

Vaidya, N., et al. (2012). "Spontaneous Network Formation Among Cooperative RNA Replicators." *Nature* 491: 72–77.

Varela, F., E. Thompson, and E. Rosch (1991). *The Embodied Mind: Cognitive Science and Human Experience*. Cambridge, MA: MIT Press.

Vazza, F., and A. Feletti (2020). "The Quantitative Comparison Between the Neuronal Network and the Cosmic Web." *Frontiers in Physics* 8: 1–8.

Vedres, B., and T. Cserpes (2021). "Network Tension and Innovation in Teams: Deep Success in Jazz." *SocArXiv*, March 4. https://doi.org/10.31235/osf.io/bpxwa.

Venturini, T., M. Jacomy, and P. Jensen (2021). "What Do We See When We Look at Networks: Visual Network Analysis, Relational Ambiguity, and Force-Directed Layouts." *Big Data & Society* (January–June): 1–16.

Vergara, V. M., M. Morgaard, R. Miller, R. Beaty, K. Khakal, M. Dhamala, and V. D. Calhoun (2021). "Functional Network Connectivity During Jazz Improvisation." *Scientific Reports* 11, no. 19031. https://doi.org/10.1038/s41598-021-98332-x.

Virk, R. (2019). *The Simulation Hypothesis: An MIT Computer Scientist Shows Why AI, Quantum Physics and Eastern Mystics All Agree We Are in a Video Game*. Cambridge, MA: Bayview Lab Books.

Virtual Reality Brisbane News (2021). "Composing Jazz is not for a Neural Network, Although It Has Been Tried." November 1.

Wade, N. (2009). *The Faith Instinct*. New York: The Penguin Press.

Wainwright, J. (2017). "What If Marx Was an Anarchist?" *Dialogues in Human Geography* 7, no. 3: 257–62.

Warburg, M. (1989). "William Robertson Smith and the Study of Religion." *Religion* 19, no. 1: 41–61.

Ware, N. (2012). "The Role of Genetics in Drug Dosing." *Pediatric Nephrology* 27, no. 9: 1489–98.

Warner, R. M. (1988). "Rhythm in Social Interaction." In J. E. McGrath, ed., *The Social Psychology of Time*, pp. 63–88. Newbury Park: Sage.

Weiner, E. (2016). *The Geography of Genius: Lessons from the World's Most Creative Places*. New York: Simon & Schuster.

Wenk, G. W. (2020). "Brain Enhancement Folly: There Are No Miracles on the Brain-Enhancement Product Shelf." *Psychology Today*, March 27.

West, P. (2017). *Get Over Yourself: Nietzsche for Our Times*. Exeter, UK: Imprint Academic.

Wheeler, J. A. (1989). "Information, Physics, Quantum: The Search for Links." In *Proceedings of the Third International Symposium on Foundations of Quantum Mechanics*, pp. 354–58.

White, J. G., E. Southgate, J. N. Thomson, and S. Brenner (1986). "The Structure of the Nervous System of the Nematode *Caenorhabditis elegans*." *Philosophical Transactions of the Royal Society B* 314, no. 1165: 141–340.

White, T. H. (1977). *Merlyn the Magician*. Austin: University of Texas Press.

Whitehead, C. ed. (2008). *The Origin of Consciousness in the Social World*. Exeter UK: Imprint Academic.

Wikström, V., K. Saarikivi, M. Falcon, T. Makkonen, S. Martikainen, V. Putkinen, B. Ultan Cowley, and M. Tervaniemi (2022). "Inter-Brain Synchronization Occurs without Physical Co-Presence during Cooperative Online Gaming." *Neuropsychologia* 174: 1–14.

Williams E, S., and R. Karim L (2018). *Physiological Psychology*. Chennai, India: Notion Press.

Wilms, W., M. Wozniak-Karczewska, P. F. X. Corvini, and L. Chrzanowski (2019). "Nootropic Drugs: Methylphenidate, Modafinil and Piracetam—Population Use Trends, Occurrence in the Environment, Ecotoxicity and Removal Methods—A Review." *Chemosphere* 233: 771–85.

Wilson, E. O. (2012). *The Social Conquest of Earth*. New York: Liveright.

Winner, L. (1977). *Autonomous Technology*. Cambridge, MA: MIT Press.

Woodward, K. (2004). "A Feeling for the Cyborg," pp. 181–200 in R. Mitchell and P. Thurtle, eds., *Data Made Flesh*. New York: Routledge.

Wynter, S. (1992). "Beyond the Categories of the Master Conception: The Counter-Doctrine of the Jamesian Poiesis." In P. Henry and P. Buhle, eds., *C. L. R. James's Caribbean*, pp. 63–91. Durham, NC: Duke University Press.

Yegenoglu, M. (1998). *Colonial Fantasies: Toward a Feminist Reading of Orientalism*. Cambridge, UK: Cambridge University Press.

Young, J., ed. (2015). *Individual and Community in Nietzsche's Philosophy*. Cambridge, UK: Cambridge University Press.

Yuan, Z., et al. (2012). "An Enriched Environment Improves Cognitive Performance in Mice from the Senescence Accelerated Prone Mouse 8 Strain." *Neural Regeneration Research* 7, no. 23: 1797–804.

Zapparoli, L., M. Porta, and E. Paulesu (2015). "The Anarchic Brain in Action: The Contribution of Task-Based fMRI Studies to the Understanding of Gilles de la Tourette Syndrome." *Current Opinion in Neurology* 28, no. 6: 604–11.

Index

About the Author

Sal Restivo is a retired sociologist/anthropologist who has held professorships and endowed chairs at universities in the United States, Canada, Europe, and China. He is a founding member and former president of the Society for Social Studies of Science, and specializes in the sociology of science and religion. He is the editor-in-chief of Oxford's *Science, Technology, and Society: An Encyclopedia* (2005), and author most recently of *Einstein's Brain: Genius, Culture and Social Networks* (2020), *Society and the Death of God* (2021), and *Inventions in Sociology: Studies in Science and Society* (2022).